Never-Say-Diet
Book

RICHARD SIMMONS'

Never-Say-Diet Book

WARNER BOOKS

A Warner Communications Company

Copyright © 1980 by Richard Simmons
All rights reserved
Warner Books, Inc., 75 Rockefeller Plaza,
New York, N. Y. 10019

w A Warner Communications Company

Photo on p. 205 by Michael P. Maron
All other photos by Kerry Morris and Steven Nelson
Book design by Paul Perlow
Cover Design by *The New Studio, Inc.*
Printed in the United States of America
First Printing: February 1982
10

Library of Congress Cataloging in Publication Data
Simmons, Richard.
  Never-say-diet book.

  1. Reducing diets.   2.   Reducing exercises.
I. Title.
RM222.2.S546   613.2′5   80-16814
ISBN 0-446-97041-7 (U.S.A.)
ISBN 0-446-37505-9 (Canada)

*I dedicate my research and this book to my
editor, Christine Conrad, to Suzy Kalter,
and to all the people who have struggled
with a weight problem—hoping your
struggle is finally over.*

WARNING!!!
Do not eat any junk food while reading this book. Certain foods will automatically wipe the words right off the pages, and the bookstore or publisher will not be held responsible.

CONTENTS

Never-Say-Diet
Book
Book

CHAPTER 0

This book begins with Chapter 0 for a very important reason. You don't have to read it. (The scale also begins at 0 and you never read that, either!)

Take me, for example. I happen to be one of those people who never ever read the stuff that comes before Chapter One: the Preface, the Introduction, the Author's Notes (yawn). All those pages with the little roman numerals and footnotes drive me crazy and can get a bit boring.

I like to give the book a good hard stare, check out the author's picture, find a nice comfortable sofa, and start at the big "one."

This book, therefore, has no Introduction, no Preface, and nothing to put you to sleep, except for maybe the acknowledgments (but they are short). So you can go directly to Chapter One without feeling guilty. By the way, when was the last time you got on a scale?

Thank you,

Richard Simmons

Richard Simmons
138 pounds

CHAPTER 1

INTRODUCTION

The only time I wasn't fat was the day I was born. I weighed three pounds, two ounces, and was one month premature. I had flat feet, asthma, hay fever, and a crummy name: Milton Teagle Simmons. It was enough to drive anyone to food.

You've heard of baby fat? Baby, was I fat. Maybe it was from growing up in New Orleans, the sauce capital of the world. I went directly from pablum to Crêpes Suzette with only a short stop in between for pralines and Mornay sauce. (Not together!) The tourists may have stopped for breakfast at Brennans'. I liked to stay around for lunch, dinner, and dessert as well.

While my peers were wasting time playing cowboys and Indians, fantasizing about pirates and lost treasure, or laying neat plans to become firemen or private detectives, I was flipping through the pages of *The American Express Gourmet Cooking Guide* and *One Thousand and One Ways to Prepare Eggplant*. While other kids were writing tacky letters to Santa, begging for race cars, bicycles, and erector sets, I blithely asked Santa for a set of stainless-steel measuring spoons, a large soufflé dish, and a copper double boiler.

I quickly grew from a smiling chubby baby to a smiling chubby toddler to the fattest kid on the block. I was laughed at, made fun of, and all but ignored. I was the last chosen for an athletic event and the first in line for lunch. I was dressed in clothes purchased in the Husky Department and was never allowed to wear T-shirts with horizontal stripes.

I discovered I was really fat when I was eight years old and my mother took me to the "I'm Afraid to Admit My Size Sale" at the biggest store we had in New Orleans. There, at the bottom of the stairs, slightly to the right of the irregular towels, was this large crowd of people, mesmerized by a slightly overweight high-pressure-type salesman who promised everyone there a new, thinner self for only $5.95.

"Don't think for a minute, my dear people, that I don't understand your problems. I've been through them myself, and believe it or not, this Magic Fingers Exercise Belt can melt away excess pounds in a matter of days."

I believed it. After a few please-Mommy-please speeches, I found myself the proud owner of my salvation. I rushed home and squeezed into this contraption made of plastic wrap and held together by rubber bands, following the instructions intently as I tied the tubing securely under my arms. Even though I resembled a breakfast sausage in it, I proudly wore my Magic Fingers Exercise Belt to school religiously for a week. My temporary thinness was cut short by a heat rash all over my back and bottom area.

The Magic Fingers Exercise Belt was just the first of hundreds of gimmicks I was to try throughout my life in an attempt to curb my weight and keep my figure this side of Dumbo's. For the next eleven years I tried every imaginable (and some not so imaginable) diet and weight-reduction method ever conceived. Even true love could not get me to keep off the pounds.

When I was eleven I fell in love with Juanita Wasserman, the foxiest girl in the sixth grade. I know she liked me because she let me carry her books once—which was pretty hard to do while eating a salami and Swiss-cheese sandwich with relish and tomatoes. When I finally got up the nerve to ask her to a sock hop, she turned up her turned-up nose at me and replied, "With *you*, Milton? Why, you're obese!"

I didn't even know what obese meant, but I was almost in tears. I didn't even like the sound of the word. I ran home, looked up o-b-e-s-e in the dictionary (luckily I was a good speller and got it on the first try) and read every word imprinted there in those tiny little Webster's Dictionary letters: "fat, stout, excessively corpulent; very fat." It was not a pretty picture.

That same day, I removed the box of chocolate-covered cherries from my nightstand, threw the cookies and the bubble gum in my sock drawer into the trash can, flushed all the peanut brittle down the toilet, and got down on my obese knees and prayed.

"Dear God, I do not want to be obese. Please take back sixty pounds and make me like other people. If you do this for me, I'll never lock my brother Lenny in the closet again. Thank you and amen."

God must have been on miracle call while I was praying, because He took no immediate action on my case. I was forced to grow up chasing dietetic rainbows, trying everything I could to lose weight as I searched for the answer to my overweight problem. I changed my name from Milton to Richard in quest of a new image. I considered becoming a doctor for fat people, or a monk—they don't have to worry about their pants getting too tight because they wear those loose-fitting cassocks all the time. Instead, I became an Italian film star.

You see, I won this scholarship to study art and architecture in Florence. I'd never been to Europe and it sounded a lot more glamorous than going to Louisiana State College with all my friends from high school who still kept calling me Milton instead of Richard. So I packed up all 214 pounds of me and arrived in pizzaland. It was my idea of heaven: everywhere you looked was a church or a restaurant.

One Sunday I was brunching at my favorite outdoor café—just the usual, a little spaghetti, a little lasagna, a little pizza, no bread—I'm watching my weight—and this well-dressed dignified, and extremely handsome gentleman walked over to my table and introduced himself. He said he was an agent for television commercials and, yep, I ought to be in pictures. A week later I was auditioning for the part of a pat of margarine, and before you could say *Mamma mia* I was doing campaigns for husky jeans, candy bars, soap, and tires. I even appeared as a dancing meatball. I was as famous as Mr. Whipple or Mrs. Olson. The Italians loved me—they thought I'd stepped out of a Botticelli painting—and I was on my way to overweight stardom.

Then I received a letter which changed my life, and my shape, forever. It was the winter of 1968. After a personal appearance at a supermarket where I was autographing gnocchi, I walked back to the car and saw this envelope resting under the windshield wiper. At first I thought it was another fan letter. Then I thought maybe the Millionaire had stopped by. Instead, it only said:

> FAT PEOPLE DIE YOUNG
> PLEASE DON'T DIE
> *Anonymous*

To tell you I almost went into shock right there, next to my little red Fiat 124, would be putting it mildly. I got this awful lump in my throat and my stomach turned into a big knot. Somebody really cared. I mean *really*.

Everyone who loses weight is triggered off by something, and that was the something for me. Die . . . I kept thinking. Fat people die young/please don't die. I didn't want to die.

I became very paranoid and very scared. All I could think about were the words written on the card, which were now indelibly burned into my memory. I quickly checked myself into a clinic outside Rome to undergo a three-day physical examination to find out how much longer I had to go. (It took them three days just to find all my parts.)

The doctors did not play nasty little word games with me like Juanita Wasserman. They never mentioned the word obese once. But they did talk about my weak heart, my high blood pressure, a kidney problem, a set of not terrific knees, and an artery buildup that would soon send me to the Sistine Chapel—but not as a tourist. They kindly informed me that I was a walking time bomb, and that if I didn't take the weight off soon I'd better start throwing three coins (or a bankful) into the fountain.

Filled with fear and *angst*, I completely panicked. I reached for quick, painless, fast, and immediate (sometimes fast isn't quick enough) remedies . . . pills, shots, massages, hypnosis, anything and everything. Nothing seemed to be working fast enough, so I quit eating completely. I tried to remain active during the dietetic changes in my life—I joined a gym so I could exercise off what wasn't falling off quickly enough. I grew weak and sick, but I saw my waistline drop from 44 inches to 36 inches and that was all I cared about. I was determined to get thin.

Two and a half months later I *was* thin. The good news was that I lost 112 pounds (thank you). The bad news was that I also lost a lot of other things along the way. Big clumps of my curly locks had fallen out. My sense of humor went down the bidet. I became irritable and began to wonder if a size "small" was worth it. Stretch marks covered my most intimate parts. Dry skin hung where nothing should hang. My fingernails were jagged and brittle. My breath was foul, and my mood matched.

I had to check into a hospital to recover from the trauma my body had been through. I needed a few nips and tucks by a plastic surgeon. I needed a hair transplant to replace my own tresses, which showed no sign of returning to my bald head. And I needed to learn how to eat sensibly. While I was in the hospital I began to read books about health, diet, exercise, vitamins, and, of course, hair growth. I soon realized how important it was to lose weight slowly and to keep it off forever rather than be a yo-yo, as I had been all my youth, or a dodo, as I had been when I went on my crash diet. I discovered the correlation between diet and exercise and the importance of the proper mental attitude, and I slowly began to devise my own plan that would combine the three in a safe, but effective, lifetime plan. I began to see myself as the Joan of Arc of weight (and we all know how many calories she burned up!) and moved to California to become the Weight Saint.

I wanted first to make sure that all my thoughts applied to Americans, so I took a job in a popular Los Angeles restaurant where I was the maître d'—a job that enabled me to see what everyone was eating without having to get my hands dirty. It took me no time at all to realize that Americans needed me even more than Italians. These guys really ate like pigs. They had positively no idea of what they were doing to their bodies and no restraint while they were doing it. I was horrified and I was challenged. I had to help them all before it was too late.

So, with a few investors, I located a warehouse and a small suite of offices in Beverly Hills and created Ruffage and The Anatomy Asylum, a restaurant with the best salad bar in town and an adjoining exercise studio. Nothing fattening was served. I greeted everyone who came through the door personally, and if my guests were overweight I'd scream "Thighs, thighs, go away, give them all to Doris Day." It was outrageous, but it worked.

Soon everyone in town was flocking to my classes and my salad bar. The overweights and the heavyweights were side by side— Loretta Young, Dustin Hoffman, Diana Ross, Barbra Streisand, Paul Newman, Joanne Woodward, Henry Winkler—they all came for exercise or good sensible food.

Sure there were celebrities, but there were also real people who needed my help. I took them under my still thin wing—the 206-pound secretary who had tried every diet in the world; the housewife who was afraid she was losing her husband because she'd put on fifty pounds; the teenager who hated her stepfather and kept eating junk food because she couldn't compete with her gorgeous mother. I put each person on a regimen of exercise, proper food, and attitude. And it worked. I got so interested in the possibilities of being able to help people that I began to research the eating habits and food vices of everyone I met. I was convinced that through the basic truths that all overweight people share I could create a plan that would turn all the caterpillars of the world into butterflies . . . or at least pretty moths.

I began questioning everyone who walked into my restaurant. "Excuse me, sir, what did you have for breakfast?"

"Pardon me, Madame, were you a fat child?"

"Uh, lady, could you just tell me what your favorite snacks are and if you eat them in bed or in front of the television set?"

Then I devised a set of serious questionnaires which I distributed all over the country via a series of stewardesses, hotel chains and addresses gleaned from the phone books I found at the public library.

I got detailed information on the kinds of foods most Americans were eating, how and where they were eating them, why they ate, and why they thought they were fat. In the end I had 72,368 questionnaires spread out on my office floor, entirely covering the beige carpet. I named them the *Weight Papers*. I had file cards with confessions on them that would break your heart. I realized that despite the fact that we are a nation of eighty million overweight people, very few of us really want to be overweight. I saw that most people had been through what I had been through but that they hadn't been able to break through their excess pounds to liberate their thin inner selves as I had.

As I stared at the questionnaires I became more and more determined to test out my ideas to make sure they worked and then go public with them. I began with test groups of volunteers at Ruffage. I received help, support, and suggestions from my internists, Dr. Hi Engelberg and Dr. Keith Agree, and from other doctors, who kept sending me their out-of-shape clients. Dr. Roslyn Slater, head of nutrition at UCLA School of Medicine, gave up a lot of time to fill me in on what's in the food we eat and why Americans are in big food trouble. I bought every single diet and health book ever printed, including the ones from the vanity presses and the private-label presses that are made in someone's garage and stapled together by the Cub Scout Troop on Thursday afternoons. I tested other people's plans; I tested my plan; I compared results. I learned what worked and what didn't work. I discovered what was safe and what looked safe but turned out to be riddled with hidden dangers. And I took in more and more volunteers to work out my ideas.

In the end, after three years of research and testing, I perfected my incredibly different plan. It's a plan I consider to be revolutionary to the diet mores of this society. It is not a quick, easy, painless plan. It does not guarantee you overnight results and instant glamour. It is not one magic potion or one secret thought that will change your life.

Instead, it is a lifelong plan that will change your life forever. It will take weight off you and keep it off. It combines three important principles that must work together:

● The right kind of exercise for your body and your weight problem
● The proper food plan for a lifetime, not just two weeks

● The mental exercises to keep you in shape from here on in

My program takes several weeks before results appear. But it's safe and it's good for you. You will not suffer any crazy side effects, nor will you go through the trauma of yo-yo. You will not start the program and then leave it because of boredom, as you do with other diets, because this program isn't boring. You will change your life forever and you will be a happier person. I promise it.

I'VE GOT YOU
UNDER MY SKIN

INTRODUCTION

It's a shame. A damn shame. Everything we enjoy is illegal, immoral, or fattening.
—The Weight Papers

The average person living in America today sleeps six hours a night, makes fifteen thousand dollars a year (not take-home), has a family, one pet, two color television sets, a Master Charge, and a weight problem. You heard me, a *weight problem*.

The average American is the proud owner of a bathroom scale that comes complete with a half inch of dust because, how did you guess, he never uses it. He has a driver's license with his incorrect height/weight there in black and white next to the color he wishes his eyes were. The average American female lies in a horizontal position on the bed to zip up her pants.

"The worst thing about my mornings is trying to get into my clothes. I practically squeeze myself into everything and then hide all those bumps and lumps with a sweater or a long vest."

The average American male just lets it all hang out over the old belt buckle.

"I'm not overweight. When I stand up I look perfect. It's just when I sit down that my stomach looks like an extra tire."

So it looks like we all have a real big problem here. Whether it's five pounds overweight or fifty, there are eighty million Americans who are currently overweight.

Some fifteen million of these are *chronically* overweight. Yet being overweight is a handicap and a menace to our daily existence; it affects not only our general health but every aspect of our life—from the job we do or don't get to the love and security we feel or don't feel.

We all know that we shouldn't be overweight, we've all tried diets, doctors, gadgets, and prayers. And we've all failed. Or, if you're reading this book, you've failed so far.

The difference is that you've failed and I haven't. I used to weigh 268 pounds. I used to be fat and round and miserable, and I didn't like it, so I found the way to beat the fat and come out a winner. And I know where you've gone wrong and why you've failed so far.

You've failed simply and honestly enough because you have never approached your weight problem and your weight loss from the right position. You have never tackled the *real* problem, despite your calorie counting, your exercising, and your dedication to new diet books and trends. You may have looked the chocolate sundae in the eye and stared it down, but you have never looked yourself in the eye and come away ready to change your life for the better. Forever.

TRUE CONFESSION

Let's start at the beginning. Before we go any farther, let's get it out in the open. Admit you're overweight. Confess to yourself that you've got a problem. Don't just shrug your shoulders and fondle your baby fat. Don't get depressed, don't get upset, and don't shove your pudgy little body under a Sara Lee delivery truck in shame or embarrassment. Calmly look at that mirror, and at your inner soul, and admit you are fat and that you are going to do something about it. Something healthy and something permanent. For yourself, forever, because you deserve it.

You don't have to be fat, you know. You don't have to accept yourself the way you are. You don't have to tell me that you think fat is beautiful. You do have to resolve never to cop out again. You do have to realize that your life can be better than it is today. I don't care how terrific your life is now, this very minute, I promise you it *can* be better.

All you have to do is stop feeling sorry for yourself and 'fess up to being overweight. Let me hear you say it: I'm fat. I'm pudgy. I've let myself go a bit. I don't have the body I used to have. Shout it out.

Now then, don't you feel better?

Now that you've gotten it off your chest, you can start taking it off your hips, your legs, your arms, your tum, and your bottom. Slap your face a few times—time to snap out of it, kid!—take a felt-tip pen to your bod, and circle all your real estate that needs some work. Grab that fat and just throw it around the room. Let it know who's boss. Let it know that you're in charge now.

COMING TO GRIPS WITH YOUR HIPS

By now your weight problem, no matter how big or small, should be out in the open. By now you should know that overeating is a slow, destructive process that continually attacks every part of your life. And once you understand that and realize that this is not what or where you really want to be, you will be ready to face up to a weight loss that will stay off. You can wipe away all those chocolate-covered nightmares and change your life forever.

You have to know up front, that there are definite responsibilities and fears involved in losing weight. You should learn what they are *now* and become able to deal with them.

For many, being overweight is a catchall excuse for everything that is wrong in their lives. If they have no friends, don't get the jobs, and can't make ends meet, they look down and around and blame it on being fat. If they were no longer fat and still had these problems, they would have to look inward for solutions, and that, my friends, can be just too painful to contemplate.

"Everyone tells me I am so beautiful and if I lose the weight I would really be a knockout; but that really scares me because what if I do lose the weight and do look super and then nothing happens? No Prince Charming? No terrific career? Nothing different? What would I do then?"

The whole world has this "what if" complex it leans on. Well, what if you never lose the weight and never better yourself and what if you continue in your race with food? So stop all the questions and the *ifs* and start facing reality.

If you are not happy with your hips (or whatever else seems to be bothering you), then it should be obvious that what you are doing and how you are living is not working. So you've got to change and change until you find the formula that works for you!

Hey, there's a terrific person inside of you—just start learning to take some chances . . . that's it, chances! Don't stop now—don't settle for anything you're not happy with—prove to yourself you can do it!

WHY OVEREATING ISN'T SMART

"You have had quite enough, Milton. As usual, I gave you extras and you've already eaten everything but the floral design on your plate. Now for God's sakes give your brother back his veal cutlet."

From day one you are urged to eat, and your personal eating habits are developed into a permanent way of life from your earliest childhood days. Can't you hear your mother's voice, begging, pleading: "Come on now, eat one little bite. Just try it. It won't hurt you." . . . "That's O.K., eat all you want, it's not fattening—so go ahead, eat." . . . "What? You don't like my cooking?" And so on. Even when your insides are saying "NO, NO, NO MORE," the food keeps on coming until you've made it gone, gone. And you end up asking, "What's for dessert?"

So before you reach for another helping tonight, here're some facts about food you ought to know.

● *Your stomach is only so big and it can only handle so much.* When you overload, you actually stretch the stomach muscles so that you are able to consume greater and greater amounts of food. As the stomach grows, so does the rest of the anatomy. A continual pattern of overeating leads to a weight gain. For some, the extra pounds creep on slowly—sometimes unnoticeably—for a period of years until suddenly they realize that they've let themselves go. Others put on the weight immediately. "I could look at a food ad in the newspaper and gain five pounds." Overloading your stomach leads to overloading your body, and suddenly you become an overeater—a fatso. You are no longer one of Them, the skinny, successful, acceptable people. And your entire well-being suffers.

• *Being overweight does make mashed potatoes out of your appearance.* Jowls appear, so do unwanted chins. Then little Shirley Temple dimples start popping out—everywhere—and then they become fat creases, then love handles, and finally tires of fat. Your whole body takes on the form and fitness of the potato pancake. "I was embarrassed at my ten-year class reunion. I kept hearing people say, 'What happened to Ellen, she used to be so pretty.' Some friends didn't even recognize me."

• *Shyness, embarrassment, and certain amounts of social withdrawal become constant companions.* "I have trouble meeting people in this condition. Anyone who is thinner than I immediately has one up on me. I feel inferior, which is a terrible feeling." Being rejected socially because of being overweight is not fair, but it happens every day. It also happens on a professional level.

• *It is a proven fact that fat people don't get hired as frequently as equally qualified less hefty people.* They don't advance as quickly and they don't make the same amount of money. They are paid less. "I'm noticing in the job market that the thinner person gets the respect and the job. I'm very well qualified in my field, but I'm the last one hired. I'm also the last one waited on in a store and the last one chosen from a group of participants for any activity." *And the last ones chosen to go to college.* A recent study by college-acceptance officers showed that of a group of students with equal test scores, overweight applicants were rejected at the rate of two to one. In other words, just for being fat they had one half the chance of going to college. Not fair? You bet it's not.

• *The medical facts.* We all know that being overweight isn't good medical practice. Fat people have a higher incidence of coronary and heart disease, high blood pressure, kidney trouble, circulatory disorders, hernia, arthritis, diabetes, gallstones, postsurgical and obstetrical complications. Do you want this made any clearer? Do you want horror stories about fat cells clogging up and squeezing the heart to death? Do you want graphics? Or do you get the picture?

◇ ◇ ◇

FAT TRADITIONS

The obsession with being thin is clearly someone else's fault. When we take a look at today's paragons of beauty, it's easy to understand how we got to be so paranoid. Thin is definitely in! Models in magazines are thin. Actors and actresses are thin. Politicians are thin and have a lot of teeth. Society, in general, is portrayed as being run by rich, happy, successful people who got that way because they are thin. It's certainly not vice-versa.

Yet it wasn't always this way. There was a time when roly-poly was very chic. After all, didn't the rich eat cake? Busty, lusty women were draped in yards and yards of transparent silks revealing a profile that looked like a roller coaster . . . and no one seemed to object. Of course, there is (or was) a major problem with living back then . . . you didn't live long. Those Greek goddesses may have had curves to spare, but they didn't live past twenty-five. Mona Lisa was a bit of a chubbette, but did she live till a ripe old age? Doubtful.

In fact, the only person who is fat and old (and a terrible role model for all of us) is Santa Claus. All year long Santa Claus works day and night making toys for good little girls and boys, and believe me that ain't easy, living in the North Pole and all. Mrs. Claus, with her rosy cheeks and permanent-press smile, spends all her time in the kitchen cooking and baking for Santa, the sixty-two elves, and the seven reindeer (how does she do it all?). Come December, Santa loads the old sleigh and begins delivering gifts. Along the way he consumes fourteen thousand star-shaped sugar cookies with the red and green crystal-sparkle stuff, eight hundred homemade fruitcakes, and a few hundred pounds of rum balls washed down by many, many (and many more) glasses of warm milk. I mean, the man is a real oink-oink. How does he even find his way back home? Yet legend has it that he does return home safely, just in time to ho-ho-ho a nice warm dinner.

With a tradition like this built into our existence, how can we fight back? Wait . . . there's more. February follows, and these enchanted little stout cherubs go right for the big red satin-heart boxes filled with chocolate—and who can forget those cute little pastel candies that say "Be Mine" and "I Love You"? Why, it's enough to make you have to have your stomach pumped! And then before you know it, it's Easter and a fluffy white bunny hops right into your life and jelly-beans you to death.

Next comes Thanksgiving, and there's so much to be thankful for. (Thankful that the table didn't break with all the platters and bowls full of food, enough to feed the Tabernacle Choir.)

Whenever there isn't a holiday season,

there are always the media. Television has introduced us to a host of charming friends who do nothing but induce us to eat, eat, eat! There's Mrs. Butterworth, the Pillsbury Dough Boy, Aunt Jemima, and Tony, the Tiger. Why, the other night I found myself drooling over a dog-food commercial. We start humming those bouncy jingles and then keep repeating them over and over again as we skip into the grocery stores and buy up whole shelvesful.

So you see, no matter what the occasion, food is the answer. When it's somebody's birthday—what is the traditional celebration? Cake and ice cream. When you get a raise, do something great, or get visited by an old college buddy, how do you celebrate? Dinner out. When you choose to cheat on yourself, do you run off for a clandestine love affair? No, you have dessert.

All these traditions, being rooted not only in our youth but in the makeup of society over generations are extremely hard to beat. They change slowly and are seldom related to common sense, logic, or good thinking.

So is the answer to do away with all these festive times? Certainly not! It is up to each person to know when to start celebrating and also to know when to stop. Tradition may shove candied yams with melted marshmallow topping in front of you, but the food doesn't end up in your mouth by itself!

If you plan on being around for the next traditional family times, you'd better stop being a turkey and make tracks like a bunny . . . for the scale.

THE ARE FAT PEOPLE JOLLY TEST

There is nothing, absolutely nothing, jolly

about being overweight. (Now forget about Santa, the Easter Bunny and Humpty Dumpty, O.K.?) Is it jolly to get up in the morning and spend ten minutes literally pushing yourself out of bed? Is it jolly bending over to find your slippers and not being able to bend back up? Are bigger grocery bills jolly? Is the four-piece bathing suit you wear jolly? I don't think so.

"The only advantage to being overweight is when you fall down; you don't hurt anything so badly because you're so padded."

If you are still not convinced (please tell me you are), just ask yourself these simple questions and then remember what Mom said about fat people being jolly. Mom sort of lied to you, don't you think?

1. Not getting into the college of my choice because of a weight problem is *jolly*.

    Yes____ No____

2. Dying twenty years earlier than necessary is *jolly*.

    Yes____ No____

3. Having twice as many accidents (fatal and nonfatal) as thin people is *jolly*.

    Yes____ No____

4. Growing up being called names by my peers and suffering hurt feelings and bitter resentments the rest of my life is *jolly*.

    Yes____ No____

5. Having difficulty meeting the kind of people I want to make friends with is *jolly*.

    Yes____ No____

6. Having unnecessary sexual problems is *jolly*.

    Yes____ No____

7. Not being able to get life insurance is *jolly*.

    Yes____ No____

8. Being turned away from a job I want and am qualified to do is *jolly*.

    Yes____ No____

◇ ◇ ◇

Now see? Erase the connection between fat and jolly and proceed (without eating anything) to finding out more about good and bad eating habits.

HOW TO TELL IF YOU'RE AN OVEREATER

Overeaters, I've noticed, break down into:

● *The Picky Ones*. They carefully pick and choose from a menu or from the serving bowls on the table, taking lots of what they like and only a little of what they're not so crazy about (so as not to be rude) and then they work over their plates with perfect method, eating all their favorites first, then their least favorites, in descending order of appreciation. To reward themselves—for being so polite or making it all gone—they then have a healthy (actually not so healthy) portion of dessert.

● *Method Eaters*. It's all the same to them. They'll eat anything. These eaters usually go around their plates in clockwise manner, beginning and finishing at twelve o'clock high.

● *The Oink Oinks*. The true oink oink mixes it all together with a piece of bread (usually the end piece because it's so sturdy), swirling the food around in a circular motion in order not to miss anything—rather like the large street-sweeping machine with its giant claw brushes that munch up everything in sight.

◇ ◇ ◇

"I just can't help myself."

"I consider myself a very healthy eater."

"I hate the thought of wasting food."

These three sentences could be the overeaters national anthem or dirge. So how do you know you're overeating? It's simple:

• When you loosen your belt buckle and pants during a meal, just to get more comfortable.

• When you're on your fifth napkin but still eating dinner.

• When you dine at a restaurant and ask for a doggie bag and your dog never sees the goodies because you ate them all on the way home.

• When you're the only one left at the table.

• When you volunteer to help with the dishes so you can get into the kitchen and eat out of the pots and pans.

◇ ◇ ◇

And the ringer is:

• When you finish everything on your plate and begin picking food off someone else's plate next to you, or even across the table.

◇ ◇ ◇

THE WHAT DO YOU LOOK LIKE HERE AND NOW TEST

This is a very simple test to see if you really are ready to lose weight and change your life, or if you're just jerking us all off. Take out your pen—you know, the trusty felt tip you just used to circle all your extra real estate—and fill in this space. Just answer this one question:

What do you look like?

You thought that was pretty easy, huh? All right, let's take a look and see. Reread your answer. Did you really answer the question? Did you tell me that you were five feet two, eyes of blue and coochie, coochie coo, or did you talk about your inner self without mentioning the real outside facts?

Of the thousands of people who answered this question in the Weight Papers, most totally avoided the question. I got such responses as:

"I'm married—very happily—I'm a Virgo—get along great with just about anyone. I have brown hair and brown eyes. I'm in sales and I wear a lot of neutral colors."

"I'm a great cook and was voted Most Likely to Succeed in college. I've held the same position for sixteen years and I read *Time* magazine from cover to cover every week."

Another group answered with other people's opinions of what they look like rather than their own visions:

"My boyfriend says I'm tall, slender,

earthy, lusty, and gorgeous. I hope we never break up."

"My mom says I'm cute as a button. I think that means plump."

Very few of these people ever saw themselves in the mirror with their eyes open. Or never really took stock of what they actually looked like. Many didn't know exactly how much they weighed—they were scared to weigh in and find out. Most judged their outer appearance by their inner beauty.

I'm not telling you that beauty is only skin deep, or to judge a book only by its cover. I *am* saying that if you don't really know what you look like, then you haven't really come to grips with your weight problem, and you are never going to beat it successfully.

Now let's try the test again. This time I want you to give a wide-eyed, disgustingly honest answer. And write it in pen so you can't erase when I'm not looking. I want to know what you really look like. How tall are you? How much do you weigh? What are your measurements? What are your best physical features? Your worst? What color is your hair, your eyes, your skin? Do you wear makeup? Do you wear glasses? Do you wear bright colors? Loose-fitting or tight-fitting clothes? If you're a woman, do you prefer dresses or pants? (Guys can answer that if they want to.) Do you bite your fingernails? Are they freshly manicured? Is your skin blemished? Tell me everything about what you look like. And no cheating this time!

THE VERY PAINFUL BUT VERY HONEST IMAGE TEST

Oh, I know what you're saying right now— "If I wanted to take tests I would go back to school." Well, that's what this whole book is in a way—

- to see what you know about you
- to make you aware of yourself
- to give you the encouragement of being the very best you can be

So stop complaining and start thinking!!!

THE TEST

(circle your selection)

1. When you pass a mirror, do you:
   a. stop, look, straighten your hair, and smile?
   b. glance as you walk by?
   c. run by with your eyes closed or your head tucked under your arms?

2. When someone gives you a compliment, do you:
   a. say thank you, you have very good taste?
   b. thank them and leave it at that?
   c. stutter and question what they have said.

3. While buying clothes, do you:
   a. adopt a style that's your own?
   b. shop for the latest fashions no matter how they look on you?
   c. buy only blacks, browns, and other neutral colors to make you look slim?

4. When you are in unfamiliar surroundings, do you:
   a. introduce yourself to the first person you see?
   b. act as if you've been there before?
   c. make yourself as invisible as possible?

5. Do you make love:
a. with all the lights on?
b. it doesn't matter?
c. only in the dark?

6. In making decisions, do you:
a. decide immediately and stick to your decision?
b. always ask for advice?
c. change your mind constantly?

7. When alone at mealtime, would you:
a. eat alone?
b. call a friend to join you?
c. not eat?

8. When a friend asks you to go somewhere, do you:
a. go because you are interested?
b. go because you have nothing better to do?
c. go to please them?

9. When it's time to ask for a raise, do you:
a. look the boss in the eye and ask for it?
b. put the request in writing?
c. put it off?

10. Do you smoke or drink because:
a. you enjoy the taste?
b. it's something to do with your hands?
c. it's a nervous habit?

11. When taking off your clothes, do you:
a. throw them on a chair to hang up later?
b. hang them up neatly and immediately?
c. toss them in a pile?

12. When reading a book, do you:
a. flip and skip a bit?
b. begin from page one and go from there?
c. read the last page first?

YOU HAVE NOW FINISHED THE TEST

How to Score
For each (a) answer you circle give yourself (1) point.
(b) answer you circle give yourself (2) points.
(c) answer you circle give yourself (3) points.

Total your score. Na-uh-uh . . . no cheating here. This is really important, unless you *like* being fat.

HIGH SELF-IMAGE (12–18 points total)
You are either delighted with yourself as a fat person and plan to enter your own body in the Rose Bowl Parade next year as a float, or you bought this book by mistake. Why don't you give it to your mother-in-law?

TOUCH-AND-GO SELF-IMAGE
(19–28 points total)
You've put on ten pounds (or more) . . . and you want to do something about it, but can't ever seem to pass up desserts or bread. You know who you are and where you're going in life, but you always decide to lose weight just after you finished eating in a very fattening restaurant. (Oh, do I know the feeling!)

LOW SELF-IMAGE (29–36 points total)
C'mon now. You don't really think you're a worm, do you? Your very sensitive feelings have been buried in food—probably since childhood, and you don't know how to become the special person you really wish you were. You're unsure of yourself and feel inferior to those around you. Go back and re-read this chapter, and buy a copy of this book for every room in the house!

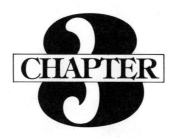

CHAPTER 3

THE TRUTH ABOUT OBESITY

INTRODUCTION

Although I had been overweight most of my life—and knew it was not a good thing to be overweight—I never really understood exactly why I was supposed to be a thin person. It seemed dumb to me to think that people might like me better if I were thinner . . . after all, my insides had nothing to do with my outsides and I knew full well that inside I was a beautiful person. (My mother told me daily.) It seemed inconceivable that I could get a better job if I weighed less—but then, was there a better job than modeling husky jeans? And yet there was this tremendous pressure to be thin because thin people had the world by

the string . . . or whatever the world is held together by.

It wasn't until after I lost my weight and became the Weight Saint that I began to understand the specific danger areas fat creates for the human body. And it was only after my life changed for the better that I could sort out the truths and fictions about weight loss and gain, health and unhealth (or whatever the opposite of healthy is) and understand how and why people let themselves get overweight.

Obesity is a really crummy thing to do to your body—it wreaks havoc on your anatomy and can ruin your sex life. There are a few other not so terrific occupational hazards:

Belching

You throw the food in, barely take time to chew it, quickly swallow, and begin the process all over again. Nice, huh? In the midst of this magical disappearing act we expel air through the mouth—usually with an off-tune sound of bubbling gas. "Oh, excuse me," you say, and you keep on stuffing the stuff in. Your body is saying to you, "Uh, could you just hold it a minute up there in production? No one is going to take your food away, so just calm down and relax. O.K.?" Belching makes your heart stop and then beat faster. You can die of belching. (The coroner will call it something else, just to be polite.)

Gas

Gas is belching of another form. It comes from eating too much, too fast, or from eating a strange combination of foods. It's not only beans that make you toot. Gas pains, usually accompanied by indigestion (next topic) aren't much fun either.

Indigestion

Everyone has a difficult time breaking down certain foods in his body. For instance, I go to a Mexican restaurant and eat a ton of chips and hot sauce while I'm engrossed in conversation and not really responsible for what I am eating. In no time at all I feel a large hole burning through my stomach. How did you guess? Heartburn. Indigestion. The black hand. (Rolaids consume forty-seven times their weight in acid.) I wonder how many Pilgrims got heartburn over a bunch of maize chips and hot sauce.

Chest Pains

"Food goes down the wrong way. Maybe it's the size of the pieces I swallow. All of a sudden I get these terrible pains in my chest and I have a hard time breathing. I have to stop eating for a few minutes to make sure I'm going to live." Chest pains are the first serious suggestion that you have a really bad problem. Maybe your eating habits are trying to tell you something. The speed with which you eat, the size of the pieces you put in your mouth, and the combination of foods at any given time can affect your health and your life span.

Bad bathroom habits

We all know that what goes up must come down. So what goes in has to come out. And what you eat, and the way you eat it, will naturally affect your bathroom habits. Some people seem to spend a major portion of their lives in the bathroom. Others pray for a weekly bowel movement. Now that's a hell of a thing to have to pray for. A clear sign of a tormented body is too many, or too few, trips to the powder room. Sure, tension and stress may affect your sphincter muscle, but proper diet will solve most of your problems in this area.

Odors

There are foods which can actually cause body odor. I'm not talking about bathroom odor or bad breath. I mean body odor. The ingredients of the food fight with the body's enzymes, and the outcome is not anything you can be proud of. Unpleasant odors actually ooze out of your pores.

Feeling bloated

You know when you blow up a balloon about how far you can go before it will burst. Sometimes you just keep blowing and blowing, challenging the balloon to burst, pushing your fate a little bit further. Many people do this with their bodies as well. They always want to eat one more bite. They know ahead of time that they will soon feel full, even bloated, overstuffed, and quite uncomfortable. Yet they are powerless to stop, to quit while they are ahead. That's because they are dumb. When your body talks to you, you better listen. (It's more important than when E. F. Hutton talks.)

DOES OBESITY HURT YOUR BODY

You bet your bathroom scale it does! Overeating is a lot like smoking. It's hazardous to your health and can be fatal. And if you think your appearance and career possibilities are hurt by being rotund, look at what it does to your innards.

People fat is a lot like chicken fat—that gooey yellow substance that you pull out from under the chicken's skin and throw into the garbage can. When the fat really builds up, you can see its effects on your figure: double chins, barrel-shaped upper arms, pudgy hands, etc. Pretty soon the fat gets between you and your future.

Here are a few problem areas that can mean life or death to you and your loved ones:

The Heart

As the body gains weight and grows in size, the heart is forced to work overtime to nourish all the extra tissue being added daily. Your being overweight scares the hell out of your heart and puts a big strain on it. How would you feel if ten extra people came to live in your house and used up all your toothpaste and toilet paper without so much as a thank you very much? Lousy, that's how your heart feels. Then the guests pour lye down your drains and I mean, you do get the analogy, don't you? Heart disease is the number-one killer of men and women in this country. Need I say more?

The Lungs

Naturally, it takes a lot more oxygen to keep a fat body going than a thin one. The body may grow wider and rounder, but the lungs do not. Pretty soon the fat starts growing around the lungs, plugging up little spaces and tightening up here and there. You begin to have difficulty breathing. You can't even climb a flight of stairs to get to your mother-in-law's house for dinner. You develop respiratory ailments and you die. You can't even have an operation to save your life because the flow of oxygen may be impeded by fat tissue.

The Skeletal Structure

Increased weight means increased work for the hips, knees, and feet. And that's no mean feat. Fat is really tough on the bones, the joints, and the frame. How would you like carrying around a twenty-five-pound bag of groceries all the time? It's just as big a strain on your skeletal structure to carry weight it was not designed to carry. Different frames can carry different weights, but your doctor can tell you (if you can't tell from looking in the mirror) when you've gone overboard.

I'm saving you a visit to Dr. Quincy, M.E., and showing you that a sweet tooth may lead to fat around heart, lungs, and other internal organs. If this picture of the heart doesn't do it, nothing will.

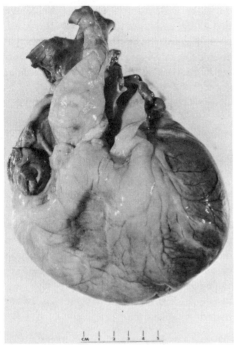

SO HOW DID A NICE PERSON LIKE YOU GET TO BE OVERWEIGHT?

I know you're a nice guy. Anybody who would buy my book has to be a nice guy. You might be a little chubby, but hey, I understand that kind of thing. I know that deep inside you're gorgeous. So how did you get to be in this predicament? Why have you been dieting all your life and never reaching your ideal weight for more than twenty-seven minutes? Why have you been forced to buy my book as your last shred of salvation and hope? Just how did you come to be fat and miserable?

There are a lot of answers to the question. Sure, you may have your favorite pat answer, the one you've been telling yourself—

and anyone else who would listen—for years now:

"I'm fat because of my thyroid."

"I'm fat because of severe medical problems."

"I'm fat because my parents were fat and this body type is hereditary."

Your answer may be a good one or a bad one—I'd have to judge them individually—but chances are your answers are really excuses. And your excuses are based on misinformation and mythical mumbo jumbo.

There is actually no excuse in this world for you to be obese. So if you'll just take this little quiz, we'll separate the facts from the fiction of your life and move on to separating you and your tubby little body from the fallacies that are keeping you from your weight goal.

THE OVERWEIGHT COP-OUT QUIZ

Reasons I Am Overweight:
(Check those which apply to you)

1. It's my thyroid. _____

2. Glands. It's beyond my control. Glands and hormones have done me in. _____

3. It's my period. I just can't help it. _____

4. It's my body type. I'm an endomorph—you know, those round chubby people. It runs in my family. _____

5. After I had my baby my metabolism changed. _____

6. I'm old, I deserve to be a little overweight. I haven't got much longer to live anyway, so who cares? ____

7. The pill makes me gain weight. But what's a girl to do? ____

8. It's my job. I have a lot of social lunches and business meetings. I can't afford to not participate. ____

9. Dietetic foods are too expensive. I can't afford to be thin with food prices what they are. ____

10. I eat when I'm unhappy; I guess I'm unhappy a lot. (Or nervous or bored.) ____

Okay, let's take them one at a time and see if you really do have a good reason for being so plump or if you're just fooling yourself.

1. A thyroid problem can lead to obesity, but only 3 percent of the population suffers from this ailment, which can be controlled. See your doctor or an endocrinologist, and then stop copping out. The odds are against you, my friend. This is a cop-out.

2. Glands, hormones, thyroid, it's all the same thing. You're just copping out.

3. Many women do gain weight before they begin their menstrual periods. This is water weight and comes as quickly as it goes with the onset of menses. If you are gaining—and holding on to—more than five pounds, look elsewhere for the reasons for your chubby thighs and protruding tumtum.

4. Body type is hereditary. And yes, endomorphs do have fuller bodies than ectomorphs. But that's no license to pig out indiscriminately. If you come from a heavy family you just have to be more careful. Obesity is sometimes hereditary, but it can be controlled with exercise, good eating habits, and a proper mental attitude.

5. Every woman's pregnancy is different. It's possible that your metabolism changed after the birth of your child. But it's unlikely, since metabolism is a thyroid function and your thyroid is probably perfectly healthy. What's happened is that your lifestyle has changed, and because you haven't adjusted you are eating at different times or in different patterns than you did before your pregnancy.

6. No one deserves obesity as a reward. No matter how old you are, there's no reason to be fat or to let yourself go. Besides, you'll live an awful lot longer if you keep your weight stable.

7. Use a diaphragm.

8. Another cop-out. You can party all you want, wine-and-dine your clients, appear as the life of the party at all the business functions you need to, and still control your waistline. Self-discipline is all it takes.

9. You can't afford to be fat. Just because potatoes are less expensive than lettuce doesn't mean it's a bargain to starch up. Use your head when you grocery shop and your stomach will profit.

10. There, my friend, may be the root of all our problems. But the answer is to find the problem and solve it—not to munch it away with a soothing candy bar and milkshake.

WHO TAUGHT YOU TO EAT THAT WAY, ANYWAY?

I was rewarded, punished, cuddled, threatened, and adored with food. Everything in my life was measured in terms of what went into my mouth.

—*The Weight Papers*

We all know that you've got to be carefully taught before you are six or seven or eight to hate all the people your relatives hate, so it makes perfect sense that we are also taught, at a very early age, to hate, and to like, the foods our relatives hate—and like. Good, or bad as is often the case, eating habits are drummed in your dear little ear during your formative years. You grow up not knowing the right way to eat and you grow up fat.

People learn to eat the way they learn anything else: subtle reinforcement. If Mom eats bonbons in bed from morning to night, you too will pick up the habit. If everyone else in the family makes gone on his or her plate, you too will make gone gone. In fact, it's a pretty good bet that your eating habits are identical to your parents' and that your figure much resembles theirs when they were your age. You may think you inherited their fat. You didn't. You inherited their bad eating habits not through genetics but through exposure.

Bad eating habits probably began with Adam and Eve. Certainly Eve had the right idea when she reached for the apple, but when she didn't get any positive reinforcement for her daring act and when things didn't work out too well in the garden of Eden, bad eating habits became the rule. All mankind began to reach for something a little more fattening than apples.

Adam and Eve obviously passed their nutritional *faux pas* on to Cain and Abel, and we all know how rude Cain was—anyone who could smite down his own brother couldn't be trusted in the knife-and-fork department, for sure. Cain then passed his disgusting habits and bad ideas about food on to his family, and before you knew it traditions were being founded that would never be broken.

If this Biblical stuff is a little too remote for you, I'll bring it home. You were born into this world naked, crying, hungry, and a little messy. Obviously you don't remember this part so I'll clue you in. For the nine months prior to your birthday you had specialized attention and womb service, then you were jolted into the real world of canned formulas, Mom's milk, and forced feedings. You didn't know too much back then so you couldn't pipe up and say, "Hey, Mom, you're making me fat and ruining my life." So you just sat back and kept scarfing it in.

Mom, on the other hand, has gone halfway into shock at the changes in her life since you bopped onto the scene and is trying to get you to sleep as much as possible so she can have a little peace and quiet. The best way she knows to make you sleep is to overfeed you. All this overfeeding, of course, is done in the name of making baby big and strong, so it's considered the right thing to do. Is it any wonder why we have so many fat adults?

Today doctors point out clearly that thin babies usually grow up to be thin adults and that fat babies will either be fat adults or will fight fat for their entire existence. This is not a quirk of nature or a piece of fate. It works this way: we are all born with a certain number of fat cells (that's right, you, me, and Robert Redford all had the same number). If the baby is overfed, those fat cells develop at an accelerated rate and provide Mr. and Mrs. Jones with one pudgy little kid. Obviously Mr. and Mrs. Redford didn't overfeed their baby, so his fat cells stayed in proportion to the rest of his development. Once the fat cells are used to being fat, there is no controlling them. Your doom is sealed. You will spend the rest of your life on a diet or wishing you looked like Robert Redford. (Or Sophia Loren, who was a very, very skinny child.)

For the rest of us, who didn't grow up in the Redford or Loren households, there's the immediate problem of a set of fast-developing fat cells and a parade of myths and clichés that only help to inflate the already thriving fat cells. There's actually someone standing over you, manipulating you to eat and eat more. Think back and see if you can't remember one or several of these ancient techniques:

The Martyr Method

"Mommy sweated over a hot stove in that lousy kitchen, slaving over this food for hours, and all you can do is stare at it. Is that any way to show your appreciation for all I've done for you?"

The Comparison Technique

"You eat more at your Aunt Betty's house than you do here. Is there something wrong with the food in this house? It isn't good enough for you, maybe?"

The Guilt Trip

"How can you leave that food on your plate when there're all those starving children in:
a. India   c. Bangladesh   e. Biafra?"
b. China   d. Armenia

The Healing Approach

"You don't feel good, honey? Someone hurt your little feelings? Here, sweetheart, eat, eat. Take more. It'll make everything better, you'll see."

Threatening Tactics

"You have until I count to three to finish that broccoli and I mean all of it or I'll burn Barbie's entire wardrobe right in front of you."

Gamesmanship

"All right now, one bite for Mommy and one bite for you. Good. Let's try that again, but this time let's swallow. Come on. You got to open real wide 'cause here comes the liver train."

Begging

"All you have to do is just taste this. That's all I ask. Please, pullleeeeese. Just one little taste before Mommy has to take a Valium and lie down."

No one ever told you not to clean your plate. No one ever said that guilt and love and food had nothing to do with each other. Instead, you are brought up with a set of food antennae that would make a Martian proud. My food antennae were fully developed by the time I was three. They would all but propel me to candy, cake, and all sugar products of inconsequential splendor. On Halloween my food antennae told me exactly which houses had the frozen Snickers and the chocolate-covered bananas, and not to waste my time at the houses that gave out apples, sunflower seeds, and dry-roasted almonds. My food antennae directed me to the kids at school with the best-filled lunchboxes, and the ways to walk home with the most bakeries and Coke machines. But food antennae need the proper environment to grow in.

Imitation is a child's way of adjusting to the world. I began to eat the way my parents ate. You probably did, too.

"Oh my God, look at what Joey is doing with his food! Where did you learn that, Joey? That's disgusting! Now Joey, Joey, look at me. Stop doing that right this instant."

What was Joey doing? Just mushing all his food together on the plate in one big mountain and attacking it with his fork locked in his hand as if it were a shovel. Exactly like his daddy each night at the dinner table. Joey's food antennae were real quick to pick on Dad's likes and dislikes and adapt them to fit Joey's life-style. What else did Joey's food antennae pick up?

1. How everyone at the table takes second helpings all the time?
2. How quickly brother Jim gobbles everything down so he can rush out and watch TV, listen to the radio, and do his homework all at the same time?
3. How sister Sue swallows her food without even chewing because she's on a nonstop talkathon?
4. How the whole family always saves room for dessert?

For the child who is observing this kind of scene at home, you know there are always too many goodies crammed in his Mork and Mindy lunchbox. You know there is a mother who buys at least one of everything advertised on television just to see what it tastes like and a kid who gets his way when he requests the foods he saw advertised on his favorite Saturday-morning television show. This is a kid who spends his teenage years eating pizza, french fries, and burgers and wondering why he has acne; a teenager who cannot attempt conversation on a date but who crams his and her mouth full of popcorn, Reese's peanutbutter cups, and other nonnutritious, high-caloric junk foods because everyone knows it's rude to talk with your mouth full of food. And this is the emerging adult who goes off into the real world finding excuses to eat, drink, and be merry when all along the only thing required would have been a new set of eating habits.

Bad eating habits got you in the bind you're in now? Maybe; maybe not. The only way to know for sure is to take this little test. Honest answers, please, and no cheating. This isn't the kind of test you score, so sit back and tell the truth. Then read the answers and see if you're not ready to change your life.

THE EATING-HABIT QUIZ

1. Do you usually eat:
   a. when it's mealtime?
   b. when you feel hungry?
   c. when other people eat?

2. Do you usually eat:
   a. in a normal eating place—kitchen table, dining table, etc.?

b. in front of a TV?
c. standing up and moving?

3. When shopping for food, do you:
   a. nibble on things in the supermarket?
   b. wait till you get to the car and start opening boxes?
   c. never touch anything till you get home?

4. When eating hot food (temperature), do you:
   a. blow on it till it cools down?
   b. pop it in your mouth and swallow fast?
   c. mix it with food that is not so hot and then eat it?

5. When finishing a drink, do you:
   a. immediately ask for a refill?
   b. suck the ice first?
   c. take a beverage rest?

6. When food is put in front of you, do you:
   a. season without tasting?
   b. ask what's in it?
   c. taste first and then season?

7. When you have something in your mouth that you're not too thrilled with, do you:
   a. remove it and put it in your napkin?
   b. swallow it and smile?
   c. put it back on your plate?

8. When seconds are passed, do you:
   a. count what's on the platter to see if there's enough for everyone?
   b. watch how much other people take and do the same?
   c. play it by ear?

9. When eating alone, do you:
   a. eat with your hands?
   b. use the proper eating utensils?
   c. employ a combo?

10. Between bites do you:
    a. chew well and rest a moment?
    b. chew and think about what the next bite is going to be?
    c. have a fork full ready for the next bite?

11. Is your main meal of the day:
    a. breakfast?
    b. lunch?
    c. dinner?

12. When preparing a meal, do you:
    a. nibble as you cook?
    b. not touch anything till you are ready to eat?
    c. continually taste and season until you put it on the table?

13. When snacking, do you:
    a. put certain amount on a plate and put the container away?
    b. eat out of the container?
    c. serve yourself a portion and leave the container out on the table in case you want more?

14. Do you have a tendency to keep food:
    a. in your car?
    b. in your desk at the office?
    c. on you at all times?

15. Do you snack:
   a. only after lunch?
   b. only in the evening?
   c. throughout the course of the entire day?

What's it all about, Alfie? Here are the answers.

1. People who eat only at mealtime (and there're very few of 'em) lead very structured lives and usually know how best to control their weight. Those who eat whenever they are hungry or have an appetite—which is entirely different—usually turn out to be blimps. If you play "Follow the Eater" and usually chew and swallow when others chew and swallow, it's time to stop that right now. If you need another face around at mealtime, eat in front of a mirror; that will influence your food patterns for sure.

2. People who eat in front of a television set gain more weight than any other group of people. If the setting is a table, chairs, folded napkins, etc., you are by far the wisest eater. If you are standing up and moving around while eating you'd better sit down and listen! They put people behind locked doors and in padded cells for moving and chewing at the same time. So settle down before you find yourself strapped to a chair in some cracker factory.

3. Please don't tell me you're one of those people who start eating cookies in Aisle 3 and dispose of the wrappings by hiding them behind the Pampers in Aisle 10? I'm speechless. No wonder you're never hungry when you sit down for dinner—you've already eaten your dinner in the supermarket! Waiting until you get into the car to start munching only shows a small bit of self-con-

trol but no class. Pay attention to your driving and at least wait till you get the brown bags in the kitchen before you begin sampling—and watch the sampling!

4. If your food is too hot to eat and you persist in trying to gobble it up anyway, you deserve the burn you're going to get on the roof of your mouth. Blowing on a spoon filled with soup so hot it's steaming up your glasses shows the sophistication of a five-year-old and the self-control of a three-year-old. I bet you're the person who eats in the car on the way home from the supermarket, tsk-tsk. The only sensible thing to do in this situation is to be patient and calm—to wait for your food to cool down and to show a little self-control. Self-control, after all, is the habit you should be developing rather than overeating.

5. When finishing one drink, be it hard or soft, you should always take a break before ordering the next. And for God's sake, don't slurp on the ice cubes or make funny noises with the straw and the empty glass. Learn to nurse your drinks just as you must learn to nurse your dinner plate. Take it slow and easy, and always leave something left over.

6. Most people season their food automatically. When mashed potatoes with a well of gravy or corn on the cob were placed in front of me, I always used to reach for the salt and pepper before I even tasted. Oh? You did too? Well, then, stop it *now*. Salt is rotten for your body because it makes you retain water weight. A little bit of pepper is okay, as is a little dash of dill or thyme. You can use vegetable salt or any of the several salt substitutes on the market (there's no real salt in it) rather than the stuff Morton's makes and be a lot happier and healthier. Or try a squeeze of lemon or lime, and for

God's sake, taste the food first before you add any seasoning.

7. What to do with unwanted food once it is already in your mouth? This is a dilemma. Many people feel that their good deed for the day is to eat whatever is on their plate, whether they like it or not. Or they think they have to swallow and smile sweetly. I would never offend my stomach by trying to be overly polite. Don't spit the unwanted remnants back onto your plate, but do discreetly dispose of them in your napkin.

8. There's no reason in the world for someone with your figure to consider seconds. Do I make myself perfectly clear?

9. Bad table manners are usually indicative of bad eating habits. Using your hands is unforgivable unless you're in Morocco. I'm not here to teach you etiquette, but if you notice that you suffer from disturbed table manners, please take a long and serious look at your eating habits as well.

10. The sensible eater takes it nice and slow, Joe. Anyone who spends all his chewing time dreaming of the next bite or minimizing his chewing efforts so he can shovel more food into the old gazoo is always going to have an incurable weight problem.

11. This is the ultimate question and one that has tremendous importance for your future as a fat person. If your biggest meal of the day is dinner, you will never lose too much weight. You gain the majority of your unwanted weight at night because you are not active enough to burn off the poundage. Unless you boogie all night or spend a few hours in a roller-skating rink, stick to a light dinner and a bigger breakfast or lunch. But be sure you don't skip any meals!

12. For people with an eating problem, meal preparation is a dangerous time. Even in the guise of tasting and perfecting your recipe you can gain a few extra pounds and sock away an extra portion of dinner and dessert. Don't nibble your way through the preparation and don't keep tasting the fixings every five minutes. Restraint is again the clue to your success. Besides, you do want to save some room for the meal, don't you?

13. Snacking is an enemy of the people. It should be against the law to snack. Many fatsos have met their demise by eating sensible meals and ruining their waistlines away from the table as they reach for a snack. If you must indulge, which I don't recommend, give yourself a small amount of the snack and stop there. Don't eat from the container and don't leave the container out for a second helping. Because it's not helping and it is hurting.

14. If you keep food any place but in the kitchen you are just asking for extra pounds to attach themselves to your body. Empty your pockets, your handbags, your glove compartments, and your stash boxes immediately.

15. I thought I'd made myself clear about snacks, but if you must snack, please use a little common sense. If you snack after lunch, you'll ruin your dinner. If you snack after dinner, you'll ruin your life. So if you have to snack, please do it early in the day and then up your exercise schedule so you can work off the extra weight.

MEDICAL PLATITUDES

When I was very young I had scarlet fever and every time I turned around my mother was feeding me. She kept on saying, "Eat, you'll get better faster." When the doctor found out how much I was actually putting away each day, he was furious and cut my intake in half.

—The Weight Papers

"Doctor, doctor, I feel terrible. There's got to be something wrong with me."

This line may get you a seat in the doctor's waiting room, but it won't get much sympathy from me. That's not to say that there's nothing wrong with you or that your problems are all in your head. If you have something wrong with you, go to a doctor, find out what it is, and then cure it. So don't give me any sad songs, because a lot of people like to create medical illnesses for themselves as excuses for not losing weight or taking control of their own lives.

Let me tell you one very important truth: there are no major illnesses that make a lot of extra weight a permanent part of your horoscope. You heard me. None whatsoever. If you have put on a tremendous (or not so tremendous) amount of weight since an operation, an illness, or the birth of a child, it is quite possible you are coddling yourself and making much ado over nothing.

If something hurts, call the doctor this minute for an appointment. If you eat because you think you deserve a treat today since you're not feeling so well, you are only making a cripple of yourself.

To understand the connections—and missed connections—between illness and weight gain, you need a little general information about the body.

Your Metabolism

"I have a very unpredictable and stubborn metabolism; it's very slow, and no matter what I eat it all goes into fat and there's nothing I can do about it."

Most people use the term metabolism the way they use the word love; if you really ask them what it means, they'll stutter for a while . . . they just like to throw the word around a lot.

So what is metabolism and how does it affect your body, your eating habits, and weight gain?

You put food in your mouth, the body then goes through a process of breaking down all the food and sorting it out (hey, you vitamins, go over there and minerals over here . . . and protein this way, please). What's happening is that the body is metabolizing the meatloaf, mashed potatoes, gravy, peas, carrots, and Jell-O cubes with whipped topping, turning all the food into usable energy to keep you going. A few people have a very fast metabolism (they're skinny) and a very few have a slow metabolism (they're on the heavy side), but the majority of us has a normally regulated metabolism. People just want to think it's slow as a reason for their weight gain. The only legitimate way to know if you do indeed have a lazy metabolism is to go to the doctor and take a test. It's a simple, quick blood test, doesn't hurt, and costs about twenty dollars.

If you are among the 3 percent in the world that has a slow metabolism . . . relax, it can be fixed. You take carefully prescribed doses of thyroid (in pill form) and your metabolism works faster; but these days fewer and fewer thyroid pills are being handed out and more nutritional advice is being given to regulate all the glands that have something to do with how the body handles food.

Water Retention

The thyroid pill (like all other pills, shots, or pain killers) may cause a body to retain water. Retaining water is another major medical gripe that many blame their excess weight on.

"My problem is just plain water retention. You see, I have to take all this medication that makes my body swell up like a football."

Swelling, or edema, is a state in which the body retains more fluids than usual, making for sore nerves, discomfort, and a lot of puffiness. I mean there's a lot of space in your body between that skin and all those tiny cells, so there is room for a bit of swelling . . . unfair as it may seem.

No matter what the illness or medication, the extra weight you put on can come off. Besides, let's take a really close look. Did the illness or its cure cost you a simple five to eight pounds? Water weight can be lost with proper eating and guidance. If you are talking about more than ten pounds of water retention . . . well, my friend, no medication or illness yet discovered can do that to a person without a lot of help from the "victim."

So face the facts, stop pointing your fat finger at the medicine cabinet, and start keeping those fingers away from the fridge!!!

The Birth-Control Pill

If you never wish to hear the patter of tiny feet, you have the option of taking the birth-control pill.

While in high school, I swallowed a handful of these pills for a joke . . . all the girls got hysterical and warned me that I was going to gain a lot of weight. I remember getting on the scale every morning praying that I didn't get any heavier. I didn't, but all the girls who laughed aloud then never stopped complaining about all the extra pounds they later put on.

"My whole life changed when I started taking those damn pills. I was always in a bad mood and I was hungry all the time and I gained a lot of weight."

Why, it's amazing how one little pill could do all that damage . . . how one round tablet can cause so many bad reactions. The reason you take them in the first place is to enjoy all the hugs and passionate nights without the attached responsibilities. Yet while on the pill, many women feel bloated and miserable and not in the "romantic mood."

"The thought of getting pregnant scared me; finally I got on the pill and ended up gaining weight. Now that I'm safe from having children, I don't feel attractive so I spend my weekends alone."

Birth-control pills can definitely fill out a few curves and account for several pounds. If you are unwilling to take on these pounds, perhaps you should consider a different method of birth control. Talk to your doctor seriously about all the possible side effects of birth-control pills and make an educated decision (a three- to five-pound weight gain is considered normal, anything more is your fault)!

Weight after Childbirth

On the other hand, if you do wish to hear the patter of tiny feet, you can't accuse the pill, so the stork gets the blame. Although years ago women were told to "eat for two" and large weight gains were accepted as a sign of healthy mother and child, a large weight gain is no longer appreciated by mother, baby, or doctor. Your doctor will tell you exactly how much weight you are supposed to be gaining and when. He will also guide you toward healthy, nutritious food that is good for you and your baby and won't put extra yards on your hips. The usual weight-gain expected these days is twenty-five pounds. That's not all baby, you know, and it's not all fluids either. Whatever weight remains after a five- to six-week period is all yours to get rid of on your own.

"After I had my baby, my body was not the same. Even after my stomach returned to normal, I just couldn't drop the weight. It's a permanent change you have to learn to accept."

Wrong. You don't have to accept a weight gain at all. If you believe that what this lady says is true, you too are a medically misinformed misfit and are copping out on your responsibilities to yourself.

You can return to your weight and figure, prepregnancy, if you want to. There are no medical reasons for a permanent weight gain. Six weeks after the baby is born—maybe a little more if you had a Caesarean—the doctor will allow you to resume a vigorous program of exercise and activity. Check with the doctor who delivered your baby first, but don't fall back on any old wives' tales as excuses for flab.

"I have had three children in the last six years, all with different weight gains. My weight gains were due not so much to the baby's actual weight but to how I ate during my pregnancies. Let's face it, the last six to eight pounds were sheer hell to get off, but I've succeeded three times—you just have to want your old figure back bad enough."

Psychological attitude obviously has a lot to do with returning to your former figure. Don't let yourself make up reasons for losing control of your body. Don't turn into a big mama without cause.

"I CAN'T AFFORD TO BE THIN"

Many people think they actually can't afford to be thin. "Do you realize how hard it is to stretch a dollar these days? I can't seem to find it in my budget to buy the proper foods for my family. The cheapest, most filling foods I can find are potatoes or spaghetti, and they're not exactly nonfattening."

Whether you make two hundred or two thousand a week, your income has nothing, absolutely nothing, to do with your weight problem.

I shop every week in the supermarket and wait in long lines with people whose shopping carts are overflowing with the wrong foods. America has become totally obsessed with convenient, tasteless plastic foods. Today's consumer is faced with aisles and aisles of highly processed packaged edibles—forget for now their negative nutritional value—that are mainly imitations of real food tastes, and they're very expensive. Why not? All those laboratory costs, drug expenses, and synthetics have to be paid for some way. The truth is that your hard-earned dollars are supporting some food industries and chemical plants that couldn't care less what was on your table, in your kids' lunchboxes, or at your sagging belt buckle.

You buy these foods only because they are so-called time-savers, and after a hard day at work you can't face the time and energy of preparing a full meal for the family. You think you are saving, but you really aren't.

"I don't have time to mess around in the kitchen. I work all day and want something quick and easy. Who can be bothered?"

So there you are, exhausted, a run in your stocking, thinking only of a hot bath and maybe a little glass of wine, standing in the center aisle of the grocery store wondering what in the world to serve your family for dinner that will be a good meal but still won't push you beyond the brink. You really wish you were going out to dinner, but that's for rich people, so you'll slave another week over the hot oven and hope the kids will do the dishes and help you clean up before you collapse.

It never crossed your mind to steam up a few vegetables or serve a salad for dinner. Instead, you consider high-cost, high-fattening foods that deflate your wallet and inflate your stomach, hips, thighs, etc.

If you have any of these items in your shopping cart, freezer or kitchen table—you are spending more than you should on dinner and wasting more than you should on food with lost nutritional possibilities.

● Precooked, ready-made, frozen prepared foods cost more because you are paying a lot extra for a bunch of people who work in a big factory cooking and packing just for you. Isn't that nice?

● If it says "instant" on the package you are guaranteed that the price of these goodies instantly goes up. And if it also says "presweetened"—guess who pays for the sugar?

● If you spend a lot of time browsing in the canned-goods section of your local market you are not only paying for the preserved product that's been in there for Lord knows how long, but you are the proud owner of a shiny tin can and a full-color label—both of which you throw away.

● If you've noticed that the soft-drink, baked-goods, and yum-yum departments (including cookies, candies, cakes, pies, jellies, cereals, and ice cream) have taken over the store, it's because these items have taken over your life—and they cost more, too.

● Cleverly designed budget food stretchers and meal helpers may seem to widen the pocketbook, but they also lead to stretch marks around the tum.

● Great advertising programs that make you remember brand names and fancy packaging all add up the cost of the products you buy—especially on canned goods, which you shouldn't be buying anyway. There aren't too many different ways to make grapefruit juice. Who cares if it's Del Monte or a store brand? If you care, you'll pay for the caring.

Whether you are a meat-and-potatoes guy or an ethnic gourmand, there are intelligent ways to balance your budget. If you are seeking the highest food quality for a certain amount of money, take some extra time and make wiser food decisions. You *can* afford to eat right. You can't afford not to.

For a quick consumer course on nutritional foods that will relieve the pressures of confused shopping and educate you on the ABC's of healthy eating, write for this *free* booklet: *The Dietary Goals of the United States*, U.S. Government Printing Office, Washington, D.C.

THE NEW SOCIAL STUDIES___

Many people say they can't lose weight because their jobs or their life-styles demand a large amount of social eating. They have business lunches, meetings, cocktail parties, and functions to attend in which they would be considered rude if they didn't eat. You really know you have social problems if you:

- Really don't have fun at a party unless you're equipped with a drink in one hand and anything sitting on a Ritz cracker in the other.
- Can't watch and enjoy a movie without a tub of buttered popcorn, a large box of Milk Duds, and a Sprite.
- Are invited to someone's house for dinner and before you accept the invitation ask, "What's for dinner?"
- Interrogate your blind date about his/her eating habits, culinary expertise, and favorite restaurants.
- Visit a friend's home and within the first five minutes after arriving go to the kitchen to see what's to eat or what's being fixed. This is usually done in the guise of "helping out."

Don't feel paranoid or intimidated, the whole world links having a good time with eating, and maybe even with drinking. Calendars were invented not only to let you know what day it is but also to help you make your social engagements. It's only when you start adding up all those Sunday brunches, midnight picnics, Chinese takeout dinners, football games, and anniversaries that you realize how dangerous social eating can become.

"After struggling through four years of college, I got my first job and started being able to eat all the things I dreamed of. I could go to a fancy restaurant and order anything I wanted. I work hard and I deserve the success."

Even success can lead to social eating, there's no question about it. But a really successful person can say, "No thanks." The will power that it took him to get up the ladder in business is going to be needed to make him watch his weight if he plans on staying successful.

The joys of entertaining and being social are many, but there's no reason why people can't get together, have a good time, and still eat sensibly.

I'm not saying that the next time you invite a few friends over for dinner you should serve a plate of ice cubes with toothpicks in the middle and a head of cauliflower with diced carrots—but if you think about it, you can switch to healthier, fresher fare.

Let me help you. In the space below, please write down your idea of a dinner you would serve when inviting a few friends over. Let's make it a guest list of eight. Go ahead—write it down, starting with booze and ending with dessert. We've all got our guest specialties that we fix only for company and that favorite dessert we don't dare make more than twice a year. Write it all down.

_____

_____

_____

_____

_____

_____

_____
_____
_____
_____
_____
_____
_____
_____

See that. Pretty disgusting, huh? Fattening as hell, and probably a lot of work in the kitchen and a bit of a strain on the pocketbook. For the same time, energy, and funds you could be serving yourself and your guests something a little less fattening—maybe even healthy. For dessert you could serve fruit and cheese. A fresh-fruit sorbet would be preferable to the chocolate-mousse tart with whipped cream and boysenberry-kirsch sauce you've got planned. Instead of liquor, how about wine? Or better yet, how about fresh fruit juices? There are plenty of good reasons not to serve a lot of liquor to your guests.

"After a couple of martinis I get so loose that I don't give a damn about my diet. I feel so relaxed I'd eat anything. Sometimes I can't even remember what I eat."

Alcoholic beverages are not the dieter's friend. They're fattening, to begin with; they ruin your taste for food and they can make your will power go to hell in a hunk of crystal and ice. Why spoil your evening and your health?

So now you've cut out the dessert and cut out the booze. What about your appetizer or hors d'oeuvre? Fresh veggies? Very good. Melon and prosciutto? My, aren't we a sport. Little hot dogs wrapped in tons of pastry and smothered in mustard sauce? Wrong. Let's try again.

As for the main course—sure, spaghetti is easy and not very expensive. But so is chicken. Meat prices are rising, and there are also other good reasons to avoid meat for your health's sake. How about fish? How about vegetables?

With just a little thought and a resolution to change your eating habits you can make merry and make healthy at any social occasion.

And speaking of making merry, many a social gathering is preceded by or celebrated with inhalation of those funny cigarettes. While there are millions of conflicting reports on how marijuana affects your health, I can plainly tell you how marijuana will affect your waistline: you're going to gain. The munchies will take over and you probably won't be satisfied with a carrot. Better to lay off the grass while you're seriously losing weight—and maybe forever.

Saying no to a cheese puff or a basket of hot rolls may be tough, but it's almost impossible to say no when you've had a little to drink or are a little bit high. The key to social eating is to control yourself and to avoid anything that will loosen your control.

SEX AND THE FAT CELL

When I was in my fat state, I didn't have any problems making love. As a matter of fact, I did it all day long. I made love to some of the best banana splits, corned beef sandwiches, and sponge cakes around. I never made it to the bedroom, for when it came to real live sex, I lost my nerve as well as my appetite.

I think my pet parrot (Cora) was the only living thing that ever saw me naked. I took showers in the dark and avoided daylight as much as possible. You look thinner in the dark, don't you think? As a friend of mine once told me, "Fat people make great buddies and lousy lovers."

Now that's a hell of a thing to say to anybody. Being overweight has positively nothing to do with your abilities as a lover. Or does it? You have to admit that all of us have been raised to believe that looks play an important role in the sex department. Being fat must count for something. Or discount for something.

"My mother taught me that looks didn't really matter. If you had 'em it just made things easier. So I'm not the best-looking person in the world. But I want to find somebody to love me for being me, not for what I look like."

Listen, I got the same speech from my parents when I was a kid. It's a pretty good speech. Dad decided to discuss sex with me right over breakfast one day.

"I think it's time we had a little chat, son. Now put down that waffle for a minute. You see, boy, I want to explain to you about the birds and the bees. Some of the birds and bees are thin and some are, well, there's a lot of birds and bees out there who are fat, and they have a pretty hard time buzzing around."

First of all, you should never—never—discuss sex initially over food. It definitely takes the mind right off the food. I know my father saw in front of him a rather rotund eleven-year-old who wasn't going to have it easy weighing so much and trying to find true love out there in the cruel world, but he could have been kinder and waited until I finished my damn waffle.

What do you say? How do you explain the facts of life to a kid who only relates love to cookies and milk?

"All right, you fat little slob, I know this is going to hurt you, but it's better for you to understand these things now before you get any older—and wider. Your chances of growing up and meeting someone fabulous-looking (with a kind warm soul), getting married, and having kids are (you should excuse the expression) SLIM. So get that body together or Mommy and I will be stuck with you for the rest of our lives."

It's a bit difficult for the parent to be so blunt. He'd probably prefer telling him everything will turn out just like in the fairy tales. Then there's the one about looks not being that important.

I happen to favor straightening the kid out right from the beginning. Let him know that the odds are against him if he doesn't start reducing. "Don't worry now" speeches usually come complete with pie and ice cream, and that's no way to begin your sex education.

I feel pretty secure when I meet people 'cause I have all my clothes on and I cover everything up pretty well, but if a romance begins, then I really panic. I mean, I want the romance to work out, but I don't want to have to take off my clothes. It's bad enough that I have to feel all those extra ripples every day. Knowing somebody else is going to touch them all makes me uneasy and nervous. When I meet someone I really want to go to bed with I suddenly wonder why I didn't stick to my last diet. And I begin to hate myself.

—The Weight Papers

Your weight will always get in the way of a

sexual relationship if you think about it constantly. If you are self-conscious, unsure, and embarrassed, your feelings will come through to your lover.

You can make the situation a lot worse by harping on it. Questions like "Am I too fat?" or "Does my weight bother you?" will only hinder the relationship if the answer is positive. And if the answer is negative, well, maybe he's lying. You can drive yourself nuts.

The answer, of course, is not to be fat in the first place. But if you are, and love comes your way, don't chase it out of bed by your own overweight paranoia. Just make sure you haven't got a chubby chaser, then take a speed-reading course to help you through this book quicker and start taking the weight off NOW.

If you develop a sexual paranoia about your extra pounds, the psychological stress will definitely affect your lovemaking.

"I'm more than aware that I look terribly unappealing in underwear and when I go out with someone that's all I can think about. I can't concentrate on anything but my God-awful bulges. My mental attitude is so bad that I hardly feel sexy or seductive. And when you're upset, you can't perform well anyway. Sometimes I close my eyes and pretend I'm one of those girls in the ballet."

If the only time you worry about being overweight is right before sex, you are in a lot of trouble. It's the same story as the one about the person who gets caught shoplifting and isn't sorry he stole, he's just sorry he got caught. If you're not sorry for the eating habits and undisciplined life-style that got you into this shape, you're never going to reform. You have to repent and be

thin for your own well-being—then you can be thin for a better sex life.

It doesn't take the *Weight Papers* to fill me in on just how important looks are when the subject is roses—or love. Sex is commercially geared to the thin of thigh and the lean of heart. If you have any doubts, just answer these questions:

1. Have you ever seen a fat person model lingerie, sleepwear, or undergarments?
2. Have you ever seen a fat person in advertisements for perfume, deodorant, or beauty products of any kind?
3. Can you think of a famous clothing designer who makes clothes for fat people?
4. Have you ever seen a fat person in a liquor or beer advertisement?
5. When a couple are pictured on the cover of a record album called "Music to Make Love By," are they fat?
6. When a new shampoo comes on the market promising you thick fat hair, is its spokesperson thick and fat?
7. When you walk into a room and begin discussing the attractive people in the room, do you ever talk about the fat people in a positive way?
8. When you get on a bus and there are empty seats next to thin attractive people and fat people with pretty faces, do you sit next to the fat people?

All around us, the beautiful people are the ones having the fun and getting all the love and attention. Do these things frustrate overweight people? ARE YOU KIDDING? You're damn right they do.

What you look like is basically a decision that you have made all by yourself. And even if you use the most convincing of excuses about those extra pounds and why you can't get rid of them, you really know, deep down inside, that the God-awful, honest-to-goodness truth is that those pounds are there because you have done nothing to prevent them from being there. And that directly reflects on how you feel about yourself.

If you don't like yourself enough to take care of your looks, how do you expect someone else to love you? Let alone make love to you?

Anyone who feels he is inferior to another person or group of people is going to have trouble making new friends, especially the kind of friends that lead to a sexual and intimate relationship. (Yes, you can have one without the other, but I don't recommend it.)

"When I go to a party with some friend or an occasional blind date, I always feel like everyone is staring at me and saying 'Look at that poor fat person, isn't that a shame? She has such a pretty face.' Then I think they are wondering how I got the date, and that they're feeling sorry for my date having to be out with such a pig like me. It gets real depressing in no time at all."

You might be paranoid. But you might also be right. Fat people are automatically ostracized from social gatherings, and the inferiority you are feeling feeds itself until you live in a miserable circle, spinning your hurt and frustration into more hurt and frustration—and more extra weight. Check out this chart:

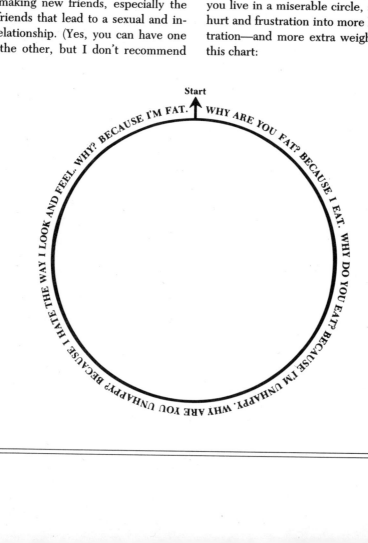

Start

WHY ARE YOU FAT? BECAUSE I EAT. WHY DO YOU EAT? BECAUSE I'M UNHAPPY. WHY ARE YOU UNHAPPY? BECAUSE I HATE THE WAY I LOOK AND FEEL. WHY? BECAUSE I'M FAT.

If you have all these negative feelings, it's easy only to meet other fat people: more overweight paranoids who are hugging the punchbowl or standing in a corner looking like a credenza.

"It's very easy to meet other fat people. You immediately know that you have a lot in common. But I'm not particularly attracted to overweight people. I can always get a date with a fat person. I want to go out with someone sexy. I'm turned on by good-looking bodies. I want to date someone breathtaking—just like all the other girls do. But it's not easy to get that kind of guy to look at me twice."

Overweight people prefer to see the beauty of their inner self without doing justice to their outer selves. If you can't face up to the truth, how can anyone else?

"One of my best girlfriends is fat like me. Well, she met this guy her same size and her same weight. Now they're planning to get married. That kind of life may be O.K. for her but I'm not going to end up with some fat slob. I'd rather never get married than have to settle for less than what I want. But I think I can do better."

In order to do better, does the plump pigeon take off weight? Oh no. He or she tries one of these sexual ploys:

Increased Personality and Sense of Humor

"My weight problem never inhibits me from meeting people, especially members of the opposite sex. I'm aware I have a lot of charm and I'm not afraid to use it. After all, I developed the charm when I started developing everything else. I might be fat, but I'm the life of the party. A good sense of humor can do it every time."

Increased Spending

If you're financially well off, you may attract "friends" and lovers no matter what you look like. "I'm the first to admit I use my money as bait, and believe me, there are many people who are just as happy with money as they are with muscle."

In the end, all these ploys are different forms of barter—you have swapped what you could have for something else in order to try to make it in the competitive world of sex appeal. It's not easy for thin people to find Mr. and Ms. Right, true love, happiness, and the perfect orgasm. Overcompensating is just another way of ignoring the real problem and hurting yourself.

THE EMOTIONAL GRIP

Overeating for emotional reasons is the worst of all possible Catch 22s. It always seems to work like this:

- You overeat because you're upset.
- You gain weight because you overeat.
- You get upset because you've gained weight.

You run through life like a dog chasing his tail—eating because you're depressed, depressed because you are eating; you never seem to break out of the cycle long enough to lose weight or keep weight off, and you never seem to find an end to your problems.

But everyone in this world has problems. Just being alive in today's complicated world is an emotional problem. Millions of people make it through the day—and their lives—without overindulging. Why can't you? That is the real problem. Most overeating is emotional.

Some people nod their fat necks and say, "Yeah, I eat for emotional reasons," and never figure out exactly why they are stuffing their faces. Others say, "I eat because I'm lonely," and continue to eat themselves into further loneliness without seeking out a soulmate or a fat friend. Very few people realize that they eat for emotional reasons and then go after the specific problems behind their eating to try to cure them. And that's why very few people keep off their excess pounds once they do manage to lose them.

If you're an emotional eater, you may need some professional help to bring your weight under control. Don't be shy. There's nothing wrong with seeing a shrink or a psychologist or joining a nude encounter group if it does the trick for you. But I happen to believe you can do a lot of the work yourself . . . if you like yourself enough and know you are worth the effort.

My parents loved my brother Lenny more than me. It's true. He was perfect in every way and always got all the attention my parents could give. No wonder my self-esteem was low. Lenny's grades were better, he never wasted toilet paper, and, above all, he had terrific eating habits.

He never ate candy, never ate between meals, and to top it off, when Lenny was nine he began growing his own alfalfa sprouts on the kitchen windowsill.

It was pretty lonely growing up with Mr. Wonderful. If Lenny and my parents wouldn't give me any attention, I would turn to someone who could love me back. Food loved me back. There was always comfort and friendship in food that I couldn't find elsewhere. The fact that the food I was overeating was making me less appealing to my peers and therefore more

lonely never entered my mind. I only knew I could have eaten all night.

Eating, frankly, was the only way I ever got any attention at all. I would purposely steal food right off Lenny's plate so I'd be noticed. I didn't pour the Rice Krispies on the kitchen floor with the milk and bananas and slurp them up because I wanted to hear snap, crackle, and pop—I did it because I figured someone—anyone—had to notice me. But no one did. So I would simply fix myself something else wonderful to munch on to make myself feel a little bit better.

We all learn, at a very early age, that you're never alone when there's food in the house. Many people can't compete with the Lenny's of their families. The lack of attention from loved ones makes them more and more lonely. Almost automatically they are drawn to the kitchen and the refrigerator for love and understanding. They never stop to think about their ballooning figures, only their smoldering insides, and they eat all the way into adolescence . . . or all the way to the grave.

Lonely moments usually lead to bored moments. Sometimes you can't find anything to do with yourself so you turn to your old friend food. After all, there's nothing as comforting as eating.

When I felt this way as a child I would have the time of my life playing with food. If Bennie Meyers and Chuck Johnson didn't want to come over and play—who cared? What'd I need them for? I had my old friend food. I could spend weeks spelling out words in my alphabet soup; hours licking the red stripes out of a peppermint stick; days on scientific experiments like testing Tootsie Rolls in the bathtub to see if they tasted different under water.

Unfortunately, these childhood ways of passing time and forgetting responsibilities grew into adult bored binges.

It's Friday night. You stare at the phone knowing it's going to ring sooner or later because someone has to call. You switch on the television and find yourself watching and not enjoying "I Love Lucy." You've seen this one two or three times before. You begin pacing in the living room. Still the phone is silent. You pace from the living room to the dining room. From the dining room to the kitchen. And there you find a can of mixed salted nuts and a Tab to comfort you until something happens. You empty ashtrays a few times. Wash all the dishes in the sink and clean the stove and realize that the phone is never going to ring. So you call out for a pizza.

Face it, a lot of people have too much time on their hands and don't have the slightest idea how to organize themselves or their time. And when you're bored you get hungry and when you're hungry you'll eat anything and everything. That's why mental attitude is so important to a serious weight loss, a permanent weight loss. You've got to know where you're going and why as well as how to get there so you don't get bogged down, bored, depressed, or lonely.

You've tried curing hurt with food and have only come away hurting more. Now it's time to face the music and play grownup. You must stop escaping and face your emotional crises head on. Don't just turn to a pile of fig newtons and demand love and satisfaction. Whatever is bothering you mentally needs some fresh air—not a bucket of extra-crispy fried chicken. Let your internal problems become verbal ones. Talk them out. Shout them out, if need be. Discuss them with your friend, your pet, your doctor, your television set. Figure out why you feel this way, why you're frustrated, and begin to look for a cure to the problem.

If you hold all your feelings inside, the only outlet available to you will be appetite. Have you ever noticed that most fat people are nonverbal? That's because it's not polite to talk with your mouth full of food. If you talked as much as you ate, you wouldn't eat so much.

Worries and stress do cause overeating. But overeating is an unconscious attempt at suicide. And I'll kill you if you die before you finish reading this book. So get your head in gear and stop chewing on the book jacket.

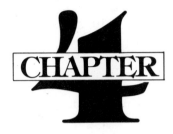

CHAPTER 4

HOW FOOD GOT TO BE AMERICA'S MIDDLE NAME

INTRODUCTION

They say sex is a cure-all, but I disagree. I think it's food. Food is very enjoyable, exciting, and satisfying. No small talk is involved, no chances of getting pregnant, and believe me, food is a lot easier to get hold of than sex!

—*The Weight Papers*

Sister Mary Margaret, my eighth-grade health teacher, spent considerable time lecturing the class on the history of the American way of eating. I learned that:

1. Hot dogs were invented in 1603.
2. Apple pie isn't really American. (Neither is motherhood or ice cream.)

3. The reason we all weigh too much is not our fault. It's the Pilgrims' fault.

You mean you didn't know about the Pilgrims? Well, here's the truth no one has been willing to share:

Many, many years ago (in 1620, to be exact) a courageous group of people set sail for a new land to call their home. They traveled through rain, sleet, and snow and finally ended up on the shores of Plymouth (or maybe it was the rocks of Plymouth), where they met this bunch of friendly Indians. Within minutes after landing, everybody chipped in and built a big table, and they all sat down to eat a dinner of Thanksgiving.

That's the historical version, anyway. I happen to believe that when the Pilgrims got off the boat, they went to the bathroom and immediately passed out from exhaustion and slept for a few days.

When they got up, they were ravenous. So when they finally got something to eat they were literally breaking their fast. And that's how breakfast got its name. The reason you eat breakfast today is the Pilgrims' fault.

Now then, after breakfast all the little Pilgrims were assigned to daily tasks like plowing, plucking, planting, chopping, milking, and building—just like the Waltons. Before the sun set, they all quit work and came together to prepare a meal by natural light, since electricity hadn't been invented by that time and Daylight Saving Time was not yet inaugurated. So the Pilgrims would "dine early" so they could see what they were eating. Dine early eventually was shortened into "dinner."

Between the fast breaking (breakfast) and the early dining (dinner) a lot of people got pretty tired and hungry and, should they happen upon anything edible (a wild turkey or a few asparagus), they would actually lunge for the food and make gone, gone.

As time went by (you must remember this) so many Pilgrims were lunging for anything they could get their hands on that the heads of the families got together and proclaimed a regular lunchtime, some place in the middle of the day. Lunch (it got cleaned up over the years) became an additional traditional meal.

As Sister Mary Margaret was very quick to explain, all this eating was as American as, well, the Pilgrims themselves. No one in my eighth-grade class ever stopped to question Sister Mary Margaret on the fact that the Pilgrims at that time weren't American at all, we just bought her theory—lock, stock, and turkey—and figured that traditions were sacred and could not be broken.

There was, of course, a lot of reasoning behind America's earliest eating traditions. Those Pilgrims—and their pioneering children—were working their buns off toiling in fields, clearing land, driving cattle, or whatever else they were doing to win the West. They needed big meals to keep them going. The advent of the Industrial Revolution did a lot to change our working habits, yet nothing to change our eating habits. Today we find ourselves eating meals evolved from traditions that are no longer viable and have nothing going for them whatsoever except the fact that they are traditional.

Societies without Pilgrims have different eating patterns and do not suffer the dietary problems characteristic of this country. The Chinese and Japanese traditionally eat foods that are better for their bodies than American foods—and they have less heart disease, fewer obese people, and longer life spans. There are people in Tibet or India or someplace sacred that live to be a hundred years old because of what they don't eat, and there's a tribe somewhere in Russia that eats yogurt (read about them in a yogurt advertisement) whose life expectancy is 120 years.

It's obvious to everyone that you are what you eat. And in these modern times if you're eating like a Pilgrim, you are a turkey.

Food has changed a lot since our forefathers got off the boat. But eating habits and traditions have not kept pace. Even as fewer fresh foods and more frozen, plastic, or precooked foods have found their way to our tables, we have not allowed a backward glance over our shoulders and into history to reconsider what and why we are eating exactly what we are eating. Food quality has dissipated over the last two hundred years. Eating habits have gone downhill. But our traditional meals are as sacred to us as the national anthem. And obesity is as all-American as Thanksgiving.

The way we eat and the way we weigh are naturally connected. Take a good hard look at the meals you and your family are indulging in and see if there isn't room for improvement.

GOOD MORNING

When I was growing up, a lot of my friends used alarm clocks to wake them for school to make sure they got up on time and had enough time to dress sensibly, eat sensibly, and still catch the school bus. Not me. The smell of bacon grease wafting through the house at approximately 6:53 each morning was enough to shake me from the deepest slumber, send me quickly into the bathroom for the morning routines, and down to the breakfast table so I could start my day out the right way: with a big hearty breakfast.

I remember it all clearly, as if it were only yesterday. The table in the breakfast nook looked like Bloomingdale's during a summer sale: piled high with incredible goodies. There was a big Lazy Susan in the middle of the table loaded down with boxes of sugar-coated cereals, a plastic bear that poured chocolate sauce in my milk (I couldn't bear the thought of drinking my milk plain), powdered sugar, granulated sugar, a tall bottle of pure maple syrup (the

syrup was served warmed up in a little copper pot on waffle and pancake days) and, of course, a tiny container of "One-A-Day Multi Vitamins."

Breakfast had a certain cadence to it that proceeded in ritualistic patterns. First thing I had to do (after we said grace over the sound of the blaring ALL NEWS Radio Station) was to drink the large glass of juice that was put in front of me.

"Now Milton, I want to see the bottom of that juice glass in less than one minute," my mother would say. You'd think she was training me for some unique Olympic event. With the juice went the vitamin tablet, then I was free to make choices within the prescribed pattern: a bowl of cereal mixed with some fresh fruit (I usually chose Sugar Pops or Frosted Flakes but always had to add some sugar just in case a few flakes or pops were passed over by the pre-sugaring machines in Battle Creek, Michigan); then some eggs (scrambled for me, please) served with parsley and paprika garnish; some fried potatoes, bacon or grilled ham, and a little toast or a muffin. We had English muffins every Tuesday and Friday morning.

"Mommy, Mommy, look! There's a few little places on my muffin that haven't got any butter on them. I can't eat those parts."

"Here, honey, Mommy has twenty-three flavors of jam, jelly, preserves, and marmalade to make it all better . . . and the tops are already off." (God forbid you should strain yourself so early in the morning.)

This, of course, was just the weekday breakfast—to get me started for a busy day at school. Weekends, when some kids liked to sleep late or eat a light breakfast and run outside to play, I could look forward to something a lot more special. The Big Family Breakfast. French toast, link sausages, donuts, cinnamon rolls—what's your pleasure? On weekends I wanted them all and usually got them all. And, if I was really a good boy, I also got my own cup of coffee—but it was doctored up so it wouldn't stunt my growth or taste icky. My mother put a few teaspoons of coffee from her cup into mine, added a teaspoon or two of sugar, filled the cup up with half and half, and stirred it for me. Delicious.

The fact that I was a little more round than anyone else my age was never equated with our eating habits. After all, we just ate a healthy all-American breakfast like every other family in the country.

Did I say *healthy?*

Of course it wasn't healthy, but no one knew that then. Did our mothers know they were training us to consume 1,500 calories a day before eight o'clock in the morning? What? You don't think the typical all-American breakfast has 1,500 calories in it? You think I'm just kidding? Well, get out your little calorie-counting booklet and look it up yourself. Donut (139 c̓), bowl of cereal (400 c), bacon (60 c a slice), butter, toast, marmalade, and everything else you shoveled in your mouth. Did you add it up yet? Not too pretty, is it? And you could be perfectly healthy eating half that amount of calories in a whole day. It's just disgusting, isn't it?

And it's all the fault of bad education and people who thought they were doing the best they could for us. Did our mothers know we were just going to school and dropping our little fannies into desks for most of the day without any chance at all of working off all that ammunition? Did Mother know she was unconsciously saying, "Eat, I want you to grow up healthy, fat, and single for the rest of your life?" Did Mom know she was pushing heart disease, diabetes, and stretch marks on her dearest of kin?

No, our mothers didn't realize any of these things. But they happened to us nonetheless. And we have only two alternatives left if we plan to better the situation:

1. Relearn new eating patterns for ourselves that are satisfying yet safe.
2. Teach our children to eat not like the Pilgrims, or as we used to, but with a new realization of what can happen in your own home at an ungodly hour of the morning.

◇ ◇ ◇

AMERICA'S MOST MISUNDERSTOOD MEAL

Breakfast is by far America's most misunderstood meal. There are people who swear that if they don't eat a good big breakfast they can't get a thing done. There are an equal number of people who say that breakfast slows them down, makes them sick, or comes up shortly after ingestion.

But the fact is you can't eat too big a breakfast and you can't skip breakfast. You positively must eat something each morning for breakfast.

To find out what kind of breakfast eater you are, take this simple little quiz. Next to each item mentioned, put the number of the item that you would eat in a typical breakfast. Then total the score.

Cups of coffee   ____

Glasses of juice   ____

Eggs   ____

Pieces of toast, muffins, bagels, or rolls ____

Pats of butter, spoonsful of jam, honey, or topping for above ——

Donuts, sweet rolls, or buns ——

Slices of bacon, ham, sausage ——

◇ ◇ ◇

Okay, now add it all up. You didn't cheat, did you? Of course you wouldn't cheat. Obviously, the higher the number, the more deadly your breakfast. Anyone could probably figure that out. But a low number or a zero score is not to be applauded. Your score should be right around 4 or 5. If it's below 4 you need almost as much help redefining your breakfast as the person whose score is well above 5.

Your body, as I'm sure you know, is like a piece of machinery. You have to keep it finely tuned and carefully taken care of to get lasting service. You wouldn't run your car around town with the gas gauge on empty and expect to get everywhere you need to go, now would you? So you can't run your body without a little breakfast.

And a little breakfast is exactly what I'm talking about. There's the right way to eat breakfast and the wrong way. Most of us grew up eating the wrong kind of breakfasts, we know that now. Some of us grew up eating no breakfast and that's wrong, too. There is a happy medium that is just right for your body and your life-style, and I'll help you find the right breakfast for you personally later on in the book.

Right now the important things to remember are:

1. You should not be eating breakfast like an old-fashioned pioneer unles you are a farmer . . . or maybe a lumberjack.

2. You should not be skipping a meal entirely.

3. You should not be so rushed in the morning that you don't eat sensibly. Don't eat standing up in the bathroom or while driving on the freeway. Sit down and do it right.

◇ ◇ ◇

Here's the way you should begin your day, so toss out your old bad habits, memorize these tips, and start your life over.

If you don't feel an improvement within three weeks, you can write me a hate letter. (Send it in care of the publisher—I hate that kind of mail at home.)

1. To an eight-ounce glass of warm water, add the juice of one fresh lemon and a teaspoon of honey. (Cheryl Tiegs does this every morning and see what she looks like—not bad, huh?) Drink this broth the minute you get up. This mixture is a delightful way to cleanse the body; it does balance and calm down the insides, I promise you. You will never suffer with elimination problems and morning dragginess again.

2. Start the day off with either a fresh piece of fruit or a glass of juice. You might as well learn here and now that you are much better off putting fresh things in your mouth. There is a gigantic *taste* and *nutritional* difference between frozen, granulated, freeze-dried, and fresh juices. Now then, not everyone can leap out of bed and run a few oranges through the old electric juicer. So if you want to buy the fresh from concentrated juice at the grocery store—please do so. Homemade fresh is the best choice, but failing that, fresh from concentrate is a lot better than frozen. And if you are buying frozen—please, please read the label.

Check for additives and artificial flavoring. There is orange juice produced these days that has never seen the inside of an orange—or the outside of Anita Bryant. Your very last resort in choosing your morning juice is canned because you never really know how long that juice has been swimming around in that can.

3. Now let's talk about bread. For years it's been very chic to knock soft white fluffy bread, which I personally ate every day of my going-to-school years. My favorite was the "wedding sandwich." Two pieces of white bread, two slices of white onion, salt and pepper and lots of mayo. Don't roll your eyes around and think I'm a sick person—I'm sure you had your own freaky combination.

Despite what everybody says, white breads do contain a few good things for you and your body. It's just that brown breads are better. Whole-wheat, seven-grain, and bran breads have a better flavor and a lot more vitamins because they are not processed so much. You can now even get brown-bread variations of English muffins and hamburger buns.

4. Certain hot and cold cereals are ideal: wheat, rye, and oat selections are an excellent way to enjoy grain and have a nutritional breakfast. Granola has reached great popularity, but brings with it a tremendous amount of calories. When you are choosing a hot or cold cereal, you must also consider how you will eat it: with butter, milk/cream, and sugar, you'll drown it in your bowl and murder your own chances of a slim waistline. These grains do have a good nutty flavor. Give them a try before sweetening them up.

5. Learn to understand the misunderstood egg. Eggs have been through a lot lately. They have gone on everybody's hate list as a major source of cholesterol, bound to clog blood lines and cause heart attacks. As a result of all the bad-mouthing several artificial-egg products have come on the market, and people have developed a tendency to turn pale at the mention of the word "egg"—thinking perhaps it will kill on contact. This is a terrible misunderstanding. Eating several eggs every day of your life is a serious no-no. Eating a few eggs a week is a good idea. Eggs are a valuable source of protein, especially good for you in the morning. Just not every morning. The yolk of the egg has a lot of concentrated fat in it so you must be careful not to overdo it. (Once I read that you could throw away the yolk and just scramble up the white stuff with a little yellow food coloring. WARNING: I tried it, and don't bother, folks, the yolks on us. It tasted a lot like yellow Jell-O.) Also, remember to watch what you are cooking your eggs in and how you season them. (Skip the butter and invest in a Teflon pan. Scramble on low heat—fresh ground pepper—a little dill, and you're all set.)

6. Now let's talk about your daily hot beverage, usually prepared and consumed before you are fully awake and aware of what you are doing to your body.

To a cup of hot water we add this heaping spoonful of brown granules and in a few stirs, presto, we have our own charming mug of hot chocolate—just like Heidi used to drink. (Have you seen Heidi lately? You wouldn't believe it!) Hot chocolate has the same properties as cold chocolate (as in chocolate bar, chocolate cookie, chocolate cake), so you are just drinking a lot of sugar.

And there isn't a worse way in the world of starting your day off. Except by adding artificial whipped cream and a maraschino cherry to the top.

If you've outgrown the hot-chocolate days, you may have moved on to coffee and tea. Not only do the average brands of these liquids contain caffeine (a stimulant which gives you a fast rush of energy, but has no nutritional value and is an addictive as well as a narcotic) but by the time you load it with sweeteners, milk, cream, and artificial goodies you are no longer drinking a hot beverage, you are sipping hot fat.

No one is going to talk you out of your morning fix of caffeine-loaded tea or coffee (in this book anyway), but do keep track of how much coffee or tea (or Coca-Cola) you are drinking and what you are putting in it. Think about trying herb teas or natural coffee-tasting drinks. If neither appeals to you, try this suggestion: save the worst for last. Follow your average morning breakfast routine, but finish up with the coffee. Don't start with it. Start with the hot water and lemon juice drink we discussed earlier, then go on with the juice and the breakfast. Have your coffee last. That way there'll be a little food in your stomach to absorb that acid and to hold back the rush of caffeine a bit. And maybe you'll be too full to drink a whole cup.

7. The most popular cold beverage besides juice is milk, and as the pretty lady on TV says, "Milk has something for everyone." There are many different types of milk on the market, pointing out just how popular this beverage is, but if you are really serious about losing weight, you should be watching the fat content in your milk. Drink low-fat or skim milk and make sure your children over the age of six do the same.

These are my seven tips for starting your day off better. If you avoid pizza and root beer, sugar-coated cold cereals drenched in cream and anything golden brown swimming in syrup, you will positively feel a whole lot better in the A.M.

LUNCHTIME

I happen to think lunch is one of the best treats ever invented. It breaks up the day perfectly, gives you something to look forward to immediately after breakfast, and means that dinner is only a few hours away. I never miss lunch.

When I was growing up, I couldn't wait for English period to be over because then I knew it was time to hit the cafeteria and get to the food. The day began to warm up as we approached lunchtime: homeroom was always a bore; algebra, first thing in the morning, was disgusting; science was interesting if we had pretty pictures to look at, and English was inconsequential because who could think of the "Rime of the Ancient Mariner" when lunch was only fifty minutes away? While the other kids in my class were trying to figure out some motivation for Eustacia Vye, I was deciding whether I should have tartar sauce or cocktail sauce on my fish sticks and wondering if I should buy a hot lunch to go with the lunch my mother made me.

Lunch was a very important experience for me. I was good at it. Most kids had only forty-five minutes in which to inhale everything tightly locked in their alligator ziplock baggies, but because I was excused from P.E. (Physical Education), I was able to put away another couple of thousand calories before history class began.

In my school there was a lot of peer pressure to have big and fancy sandwiches and a lot of change in your pockets to spend on all the candy machines that lined the recreation area. *Everyone* ate crummy lunches, and was proud of it. Even if Mom packed you the most simple of foods, you soon embellished by trading or buying from the vending machines.

In the few years that it's been since Cor-Jesu High School, I haven't seen much change in kids' lunches. Tradition has rooted us in bologna sandwiches with extra mayo, a package of chips, and an imitation fruit drink. Now don't tell me you send your kids to school with a container of yogurt and a peach because I won't believe you. Or if you really do send them to school like that, don't tell me they don't trade with other kids for a certain quantity of junk food.

The other day I overheard a mother giving her child a little motherly advice as they approached the schoolyard. "If I catch you giving or throwing away this apple, you'll be in a cast up to your neck until Christmas."

What a charming way to teach little Ronnie Sue the benefits of nutrition! From personal experience I can tell you that threats will never work and the oranges, apples, and bananas never end up in the kid's mouth.

Since most children don't practice good eating habits, it's not unreasonable that they grow up to be adults with bad eating habits. From munching Fritos from our Roy Rogers/Dale Evans lunchboxes we become adults who fall into equally disastrous, and fattening, eating patterns, which become a way of life.

From the *Weight Papers* I was able to see several distinct lunchtime eating patterns that many Americans indulge in that are indicative of poor planning and big hips. See how many of these lunchtime sins you have committed recently:

Refrigerator Perusal

People who eat lunch at home often play American's favorite noontime game—open the fridge. They stand there wrapping and unwrapping bowls of leftovers, nibbling away as they take inventory of the goodies accumulated during a week's bad eating. By the time they've decided what to warm up for lunch, they've eaten a piece of meatloaf, a carrot, a few old olives, and some cold baked beans.

Thou Shalt Never Raid the Refrigerator Indiscriminately

Leftover toting: bringing the leftovers you should never have eaten while you were perusing the fridge to work with you for lunch is as great a sin as staying at home and stuffing yourself. Come to think of it, it's a bigger sin. At home you may eat something sensible. Once it's packed into your neat little brown lunchbag you're stuck with it and you're going to eat it.

Many people who bring their lunches to work with them do not plan ahead. They pack whatever they see in the refrigerator and are forced to take what's there. (Spaghetti and meatballs do make a messy sandwich, true, but it has been done.)

You don't have to eat a string-bean sandwich and a grape soda for lunch. You can take something good to eat—and good for you—if only you think about it. Lunch containers have been redesigned recently so you can bring yogurt, cottage cheese, water-packed tuna—whatever you want—to eat at your desk or in the cafeteria without ruining your health and your figure. Just be sure not to drown the sensible foods in dressings and gravies.

Thou Shalt Not Take Fattening Leftovers to Work with You for Lunch

Indiscriminate dining out: most people eat a lunch that has been prepared by someone else (and I don't mean Mom) either in a restaurant or from a food truck. Whether people drive up for lunch at a fast-food franchise, phone down to a deli or hamburger-delivery joint, or go out on an expensive-expense account feast, they all sin the same way. Whatever their reasons and excuses, they just don't choose sensible foods.

Sometimes they are on business lunches in which hiring or firing may be taking place; maybe they are celebrating a co-worker's engagement or promotion; perhaps they are just stepping out to eat lunch as a means of escape from a boring job. Whatever the reason, the result is almost always the same. Lunch is chosen for the wrong reasons, consumed the wrong way, and becomes part of your thighs and upper arms in approximately two days.

You *can* eat out sensibly, have a good time and still not add weight to your frame. Later in this chapter I'll tell you exactly how.

But remember, thou shalt eat out care-fully.

DINNER

Dinner is everybody's favorite meal of the day: whether people skip breakfast, indulge at lunch, or fast all day they're always ready to eat when it gets to be dinnertime. So it's no surprise that more unnecessary weight is gained at dinner than at any other meal.

Dinner is usually the social event of the day. It may be a dinner date or a family dinner where everyone gets together to talk about what he did that day, but it's almost always the main event.

The typical American family sits down to a meal that looks something like this:

- Bread, biscuits, or rolls, and butter
- A small salad with several bottled dressings scattered around the table OR a lime Jell-O mold with canned fruit cocktail mixed inside OR (on days when no one remembered to pick up a head of lettuce) a can of soup
- Chicken, fish, or meat—fried, boiled, baked or barbequed, and usually served with some sort of gravy made from grease drippings or sauce from a bottle or package
- Rice, OR potatoes, OR pasta, OR a noodle casserole with butter, sour cream, and melted cheese to add a little flavor
- One vegetable (frozen or canned, rarely fresh) served with a mystery sauce invented to disguise the real taste of the vegetable
- Dessert, which usually isn't fresh fruit and usually is some kind of baked goods like cake, pie, or cookies which really don't taste very good unless they have ice cream on top of them

If it sounds disgusting to you, take a look at your dinner table tonight. Is the meal your family is eating healthy or is it just all-American.

I came from one of those all-American families that associated the amount of food with material success and good living. Not only was there a lot of food served in our household, but it was served in a sumptuous manner. Even good healthy foods, when they were served, were smothered in sauces, gravies, or accessories clearly un-called-for at any event other than a baccha-nalian feast.

Salads. "I need the croutons and the ground pepper, oh, and some more dressing, my salad's too dry. Any Parmesan cheese in the house? And don't put beets in my salad again, all right? I hate red things in my sal-ad."

Main Protein (meat, fish, or fowl). "Where's the A-1 sauce? (Or the garlic salt and Worcestershire stuff for the steak.) Are we out of ketchup? This fish is fishy. Can you pass me the tartar sauce? I don't want a spoonful, give me the jar, this is a big piece of fish. This chicken dish is flat-tasting. I think it needs more salt. This hamburger (hot dog) is lonely for some onions, relish, mustard, mayonnaise and hot sauce."

Starch. "Yes, everything on the potato, yes, everything—sour cream, bacon bits, butter, chives, salt and pepper. Mush it all up and then melt some cheese on the top—lots of cheese. O.K. I need some salt for the french fries—it cuts the grease, you know. Ketch-up, too, please. Who forgot to butter the noodles? They're terrible. Why didn't you add that can of cream-of-mushroom soup to the rice like I asked you? If I wanted plain rice, I could have gone to a Chinese restau-rant. I need more sauce on my spaghetti and some cheese and red-hot crushed pep-pers—that's the way to eat spaghetti!"

Vegetables. "Hurry up, I like to butter, salt,

and pepper my corn while it's hot. Give me a break. You know I can't eat asparagus with-out Hollandaise sauce—I hate the taste of asparagus. Why didn't you fry the eggplant like you always do? Take this stuff off my plate, I'm getting sick."

Dessert. "Oh my God, this is heaven, just heaven, but it could use a small dollop of ice cream. And could you put some more whipped cream on these strawberries? They're really very sour this year. If you think that cake tastes good now, stick it in the microwave and then put some hot marshmallow sauce on it. You won't believe it."

Like lunch, dinner has become a form of en-tertainment. Seeing how much you can stuff into your mouth while still sitting up could probably get you a TV special. How did this happen?

I'm not really sure. But as the family stopped communicating, or as television re-placed conversational art, eating became a good way to fill in the gaps. Or maybe all our parents who either came from the old country or lived through the Depression (or both) just didn't ever want to see their chil-dren sit at a table that wasn't laden with enough food for a week. Whatever the causes, obesity is the result.

It's all right to have dinner as the princi-pal event of the day—for people to get to-gether and swap ideas or, you should excuse the expression, chew the fat—but they don't have to keep eating while they're being en-tertained. Dinner should be the lightest of the day's three meals because you are the least active after you eat it. Dinner can be the climax of the day, but it should be healthy.

SNACKING

It's 1743. Chocolate-chip cookies continually disappear from a large glass apothecary jar in the pantry. Nobody will admit to the crime. Late one night, Sir Robert Cherryhill hides under the stairwell, his eyes closely watching the jar. . . . Suddenly, light footsteps slowly make their way down the stairs to the pantry. Sir Robert quickly lights a candle and shouts, "Stop, thief—they are mine! I've caught you in the act and you will be snacked . . . I mean smacked."

With amazement Sir Robert discovers the offender is none other than his fair wife, Martha, who is with child and hungry in the middle of the night for milk and cookies. Martha became the first official snacker in history (if you discount Eve).

The urge to snack comes without warning. You can be minding your own business, reading a magazine, cleaning out a closet, and suddenly it comes upon you. You don't think you can go another minute without:

a. a brownie;
b. an ice-cream cone;
c. a chocolate-covered caramel bonbon or two, or three, or four.

Your will power dissolves to naught. You are a slave to this whim. You'll simply die if you don't satisfy yourself instantly, and despite all your dieting or careful meal planning, you suddenly find yourself five pounds heavier—or fifteen or fifty!!! Snacking can do you in.

"I used to sneak in the kitchen and stuff Nabisco Chocolate Mallomars in my bra (covered up with a big robe so my husband wouldn't notice), rush into the bathroom,

turn on the water or blow dryer, and eat them until I couldn't move."

Whether you hide or do it where everyone can see, snacking is a universal problem. If you could stop it cold turkey, you would be saving yourself more than ten pounds a year in extra weight. But since that's probably impossible for most, I'm including some snacking suggestions that can come in handy.

● Try to keep your house free from fattening foods. Start saving pennies in your cookie jar . . . grow a plant in the candy dish. I always have a large container in the fridge filled with radishes, cauliflower, string beans, celery, carrots, and, of course, water—that way they remain ice cold and very crunchy (snackers love to hear things make noise in their mouth).

● Now you're wondering what to keep in the freezer section when you get crazed for something icy! Frozen grapes (seedless)—you heard me, frozen grapes—they work every time. Just wash, clean, and remove them from the stems and place them in the freezer. When you just gotta have something in your mouth, pop a frozen grape in there. As you roll it around your mouth waiting for it to thaw (twenty to twenty-five minutes), you get a sweet, refreshing sensation. Don't laugh at the idea, try it. (Sure beats sucking on a sour pickle, and I known a lot of snackaholics who do just that!)

● When you're at a double feature and you run out to the lobby, buy a small popcorn without the butter (or the stuff that looks and tastes like butter). Eat it one kernel at a time—it lasts longer that way. Pass on the Milk Duds, strawberry licorice, and ice cream. Don't bring apples with you to the theater—they're too noisy, and where do you hide the core? Forget it, don't tell me.

● Going to other peoples' houses for a party or a small informal get together is the hardest time because, you see, they are also watching their weight and they serve all the junk they have in the house so they don't have to face it every day. I used to throw the food on the floor and announce to one and all that they didn't need to eat the chips and miniature egg rolls and hot dogs and I was doing them a great big favor. (Wasn't invited to too many other parties after that.) What I always do now when I'm out and about and food is staring at me is try to find the lesser of the evils and have a small portion of it. I stay away completely from bowls of peanuts (roasted or salted) and bridge mix and usually head for the cheese and crackers and raw vegetables.

● The office is still another place where snacking is a natural. Those that you work with are always bringing in tempting home-made goodies and shoving them right under your nose. Make up your mind—do you want snacks or do you want lunch?—because both are out of the question. Don't keep food in your desk drawers or a container of mints in your office (for clients, of course) 'cause you'll end up minting yourself till they're all gone. It's not easy to say no to snacking, but so far has any of the bad eating habits we have been easy to break? You must think of snacking as just another meal and learn to control those times when loneliness, boredom, and depression start to take over. Remember, there is *nothing* healthy about being overweight, even if all your snacks are healthy ones.

EATING OUT_____

Everyone seems to agree that dining at home isn't really the big problem—it's dining out that presents so many temptations you can't possibly say no to. Here are just a few situations that our waistlines have to put up with:

● *You're the Guest:* You've just been invited to the boss's house to meet the family and eat his wife's specialty dishes. Dare you explain about your diet?
● *Potluck Dinners:* Your best friend insists that you come for a casual little dinner . . . deep-dish pizza, fried shrimp, onion rings, baked beans, and a little of anything else that happens to be in the back of the fridge. No salad is served that might substitute for your meal. Do you starve?
● *Family Visits:* It's reunion time. Aunt Tillie and your mom have been cooking up a storm. Dare you offend them by not tasting everything and having seconds?
● *Fancy Dining:* You arrive at Le Très Chic right on time. They have a six-page wine list and a menu that looks like a Russian novel. Can you just order a shrimp cocktail and still have a great time?

Believe it or not, you should be able to eat out—at friends' or in a restaurant—and not regret it. You'll need to speak up and make your situation perfectly clear—preferably at the time of the invitation, not at the time dinner is being served. Volunteer to bring your own food with you (Carol Channing does, and she still gets invited to the nicest places). Suggest that the hostess fix you a simple salad with a lemon-vinegar dressing. If need be, just pick at the food on your plate without going too far to be polite or join the clean-plate club. And remember these simple rules:

◇ ◇ ◇

HOW TO EAT OUT AND NOT PIG OUT

1. Make sure the restaurant chosen has something you can eat. Don't just go along with the gang to Colonel Sanders when you really don't feel like chicken or ribs but don't want to speak out!

2. Now the next one's a little odd, but it has saved me from a lot of extra pounds. Go to the bathroom before sitting at your table. Now, once you're in there start washing your hands and look in the mirror right in front of you (unless, of course, you really have to go to the bathroom; do that first and then wash your hands). Seriously, look at that mirror and ask yourself, "How hungry am I? Not that hungry really. Good, then behave yourself when that menu comes. O.K.?" (Please talk to yourself mentally, not verbally; someone may think you're a little nutsy and report you to the owner.) This is a lesson in cultivating food control.

3. If you had a late breakfast or large lunch and you don't feel like eating, then don't eat. Order a beverage (no, not champagne and orange juice) and talk a lot. Or get a scoop of cottage cheese. Play with the straws; stack the sugar cubes; rearrange the tables. Keep busy. If you're dining alone, bring a book and feed your brain—it's not fattening!

4. If you just feel like a light meal, order one. Don't get tempted by the food you see around you or what your tablemates are ordering. If all you want is a shrimp cocktail ("May I have my cocktail sauce on the side,

please? Thank you."), order it and don't feel obligated to have anything more.

5. If you are really ravenous (which is a term you should use only if you've been on a safari or five days without food and water), you'll need to calm down and go right in that bathroom again. Obviously the first time didn't work. Look in the mirror and say, "I am not ravenous, I had a nice breakfast and I am watching my weight. I am being childish and emotional and will regret eating a big lunch when I return to work." Splash a little cold water on your face, smile, and you'll be just fine.

DIETING

One of the reasons Americans weigh so much is that they're always on diets. It's true. But the diets never work—in fact, they have reverse results. After you've obeyed the strictures of the diet you give yourself a treat—a 2,300-calorie treat. Or, once you've lost your desired weight, you bask in the glory of your new beauty for a week and then begin to cheat. You gain more weight than you lost. You do terrible disservice to your body. You yo-yo your life away in a miserable eating game that can ruin your health.

Take a look in your local bookstore. The country has gone diet-crazy. Every week there seem to be fifty new diet, exercise, or beauty and health books all geared to make you stay thin forever. Each magazine on the newsstand offers you the same hope as it prints diet after diet: the sex diet, the movie-star diet, the protein diet, the carbohydrate diet. My favorites are the diets you can send away for and the reducing plans that come from mail-order post-office boxes.

"Desperate housewife who has tried

countless diets and failed reveals an amazing new diet that she discovered while climbing the African mountains. That's right, folks, she risked her life to bring you these weight-loss secrets of the pygmies and now they can be yours [the secrets, or the pygmies?] if you send your check or money order for $10.95. Please hurry, this offer is limited."

So we snip coupons, rip off box tops, and send away for these colorful books and pamphlets that promise us a "fast and safe weight loss with visible difference in twenty-four hours."

Did I send away for all this junk when I was overweight? Absolutely. As a matter of fact, I had so many gadgets, diet books, and magic potions that I could have opened up my own retail store. And most of the people who answered my questionnaire also admitted to the same:

"You name it and I've bought it and tried it. Every time I bring a weight-loss plan home, my husband throws a fit. The other day he said to me, 'Joan, by the time you're ready to die, you'll be the leading authority on food and diet and still have ten pounds to go.' "

DIET BY NUMBERS

One of the most popular methods of dieting is based on the theory that if you keep a good count on what you are eating, you can control your weight. These diets usually rule out the intake of certain foods (because they are high in whatever it is you are counting) and emphasize the food you are told by the creators of the diet to eat. Most of these diets are very strict and make it perfectly clear that "this diet will not work if you are eating anything, I mean anything,

not allowed." Even a teeny-weeny taste, a crumb or a smidgen, will throw you off, and the perfectly designed system will crumble at your feet, leaving you fat and worried, ready to start over in an effort to do better next time.

After you get all the do's and don't's down, these diets will tell you about the fancy clinics that used their diet on five hundred women who were considered hopeless, yet after several months on this particular diet, they lost all the extra weight, got married to a doctor (or a lawyer), and went back to college to get a Ph.D.

You are manipulated to believe that if these patients can lose the weight and change their lives, so can you, and you can't wait to begin any number of counting diets.

Like the CALORIE-COUNTING DIETS. You've heard the word "calories" for years, and you know it has something to do with gaining weight because all food contains calories. You study up on it and discover that one pound equals approximately 3,500 calories (that's an awful lot of calories) and you decided to diet accordingly.

You immediately buy one of those books that tells you how many calories are in every food ever invented and you begin looking up your favorite foods and memorizing numbers. It gets more depressing by the second. You look at the chart they give you for what you are supposed to weigh—according to your height and build—and discover you should lose twenty pounds. That's 70,000 calories too many you have already socked away with no way of recovery.

With the little book by your side and your sample menus tacked to the refrigerator, you begin to rearrange and reevaluate your eating habits. You discover that in an average day you are putting away thousands of calories. But wait, don't despair, guess what? Your body burns up calories all day long, and fat, which is considered fuel, gets burned up with every movement and action you take. Your body actually burns up calories when you're asleep. It burns up more calories when you climb stairs, mow the lawn, or jog.

So the secret to this kind of diet is to cut down the number of calories you eat and increase the number of calories you burn off.

The Mayo Clinic received a lot of attention and press for their famous calorie-counting diet. This diet became one of those fads that was imitated all over the country, and for a while millions of people were preoccupied with figuring out how many calories were in certain foods and whether they were allowed to partake or not.

"Everything I like either had too many calories in it or wasn't considered food for the diet. I knew certain things were nutritious and healthy for me, but when I looked them up in the calorie counter and saw how many calories were in them, I didn't have the heart to eat them. I got very bored and couldn't make sense out of it—if it was the number of calories or the quality of the food or if you burned them all off."

Then there's CARBOHYDRATE COUNTING. You just stop counting calories and substitute the same method with carbohydrates. This nutrient group is primarily made up of sugars and starches, which are chief blubber makers—but do provide the body with pure energy. The carbohydrate diet counting method allows you to eat all you want of certain foods while curtailing your intake of other foods now measured by grams. In or-

der to lose weight, you must reduce your daily carbohydrate intake to between fifty and sixty grams, which isn't a lot when you consider that there are fifty grams of carbohydrates in eight apricots. So here you go again with the pad and the pen, adding up your score for the day.

"I did lose some weight on the low-carbohydrate diet, but I didn't feel good when I was on it. I was always kind of tired and nauseous. I felt light-headed and weak and I even blacked out a few times. I really missed the foods I wasn't allowed to eat."

One step beyond these two diets is the combination of the two, which is commonly known as the CARBO-CALORIE DIET. It's a very easy way of measuring, multiplying, and dividing the food you are going to eat. But unless you are good in mathematics, algebra, and trigonometry, you may be in overweight trouble. As it says in the beginning of the book, "A little mistake can wipe you out for the whole day."

After the COUNTING DIETS come the PROTEIN DIETS. You don't have to count up little proteins all day long, so it's a lot easier than some of the previously mentioned weight-loss plans. In fact, on these diets there are certain foods that you can eat as much of as you want to, and they are usually proteins.

The STILLMAN DIET, named for Dr. Robert Stillman, is one of the most popular protein diets. First, you cut out all sugars and starches. You live just on lean meats and poultry, fresh fish and seafood, eggs, low-fat cheese, and drink plenty of liquids—eight glasses of water per day, in addition to black coffee, tea, and sugar-free soda pop.

"One thing is for sure, I spent a lot of time urinating when I was on the Stillman

Diet. Just for the hell of it I wanted to dip a piece of steak into hot fudge sauce. I was dying to cheat."

The ultimate COUNTING DIET is the DR. ATKINS DIET, where you get to count fat! This is the fat vs. fat diet, the idea being that by eating lots of the right kind of fat, you set the already stored-up fat into motion and it just slides off your thighs. The new fat stimulates body production, which releases all the fat that has been just sitting around making you look bad. On the ATKINS DIET you can eat salads made with mayonnaise, lobster with butter sauce, bacon, and many other fatty foods. Sugars and starches are not allowed, only proteins and fats. A lot of doctors disagreed with Dr. Atkins and said too much fat created too high cholesterol levels, which lead to too many heart attacks, so the diet became very controversial.

Dr. Herman Tarnower (Mr. Scarsdale) and Nathan Pritikin (not a doctor but an engineer turned director of the California Longevity Center) tried combining and simplifying the whole counting game with their much publicized and very strict diets.

Pritikin devised a plan to help people who were prime candidates for strokes and heart attacks. Instead of surgery and its complications, all you had to do was fly to Santa Barbara (now located in Santa Monica, California), stay thirty-one days, spend around four thousand dollars, and get a whole lot better without ever seeing an operating room. You would, though, have to go through test after test, walk after walk, and learn to eat a brand-new way. Nathan's middle name should have been *no*, because that's exactly what he preaches: *no fats, no oils, no salt, no cholesterol, no coffee,* and *no tea*. Once you left the clinic you pretty much had to stay with all of these no's or the problems you had with your health would return.

Due to the success of the work, Nathan and friends wrote books and related recipes for the "Live Longer Now Diet."

What Nathan Pritikin does every day of his life to save clogged arteries and "over the border" souls is miraculous—his diet, on the other hand, is monotonous.

Although the SCARSDALE DIET has been around for many years (nineteen, to be exact), it didn't really reach its peak until it became chic. I received a copy of his program through the mail three years ago from a fashion editor in New York who wrote, "This is the very 'in' diet and anyone who's anyone is going Scarsdale."

The sheet with the diet rules and exact menu had been Xeroxed so many times it looked as though it had been through two wars. There were no substitutions or additions; breakfast was the same every morning: grapefruit, 1 slice of dry protein bread toasted, coffee or tea (you're a far better person than I if you can face a grapefruit every morning). Lunch and dinner varied, but were rigid. "In" restaurants began adding the Scarsdale Way to their menu (now if that ain't chic, I don't know what is).

It really doesn't matter what you're keeping track of: calories, proteins, fats, carbohydrates, or someone's idea of the perfect disbursement of all of the above. You are still looking for a magic formula to solve a problem that really needs a sensible solution. People usually lose interest in a diet after a while—they need a plan for their whole lives that they are comfortable with, not a lot of numbers and rules that are so strict they feel miserable.

DING-DONG DIETS

As dieting becomes more and more popular and diet books and products prove to sell well in the marketplace, more and more people come up with their own versions of how you should be eating. Some of these methods are highly imaginative and follow unbalanced and crazy methods of eating—or not eating.

A day doesn't go by that someone doesn't come into my restaurant and ask me about some freaky diet she read about at the beauty shop or heard about while eavesdropping on a conversation in an elevator. For the most part, these diets are unsafe, unnutritious, and unsound and should be avoided. If you do happen to lose some weight on them, I'm afraid you've lost it in your mind and not around your middle.

My all-time favorite is the one a model told me about: it's called the MELLOW JELL-O DIET. All you eat is Jell-O and cotton balls for a week. Jell-O and cotton balls, you may ask, as I did. Oh, yes. The cotton balls fill you up so you're not hungry (and they come out in the toilet the next day) and you get real skinny, real fast.

Then there's the SUCK AND SHUCK DIET. This is the one where you suck on a lemon slice before each meal. That's supposed to take away your appetite so you will eat less and therefore lose weight. It makes me sick.

What about the MONO-FOOD DIETS. You get to eat all you want of one food. Bananas, lollipops, hot dogs, peanut-butter sandwiches, even booze. All you do is eat this one food, three times a day, and nothing else. Need I tell you how dangerous this diet is?

"I decided on an ice-cream sandwich. I loved them and confessed to a friend of mine that I could live on them. So I ate one for breakfast, one for lunch, and one for dinner. I thought this diet made a lot of sense because of the 'body confusion theory.' You know, your body gets confused by eating too many foods and can't handle it all so it has trouble synthesizing and you gain weight. Eating only one thing cleans out your body and helps it run better. Or so I thought. And your body has more time to burn up your extra fat. I got awful sick and haven't eaten an ice-cream sandwich in about two years."

The "body confusion theory" is false. There's no such thing, and don't let anyone try to tell you there is. Even the famous RICE DIET, which has been around for hundreds of years, allows you to eat more than just rice.

The degree of your well-being and the number of years you plan to live greatly depend on the many foods your body needs. If you don't provide this variety of foods, you will get sick and die. End of story. And you won't even die skinny.

Another ding-dong diet I like a lot is based on counting the number of chews. A young gentleman came into my restaurant and made himself a large salad. He sat at a table in the back, took out a little black box which he held up to his ear, and then flicked a switch. I watched him take a bite and chew it a certain number of times while he carefully watched the little black box. I invited myself over to his table and said, "May I ask what you're doing? Didn't I see one of those little black boxes in the last James Bond movie?"

The young man explained to me the "Chew Theory of Life." He believed that if he chewed each mouthful one hundred times, it would help him to lose weight. Now I agree that proper chewing of your food is very important to digestion and elimination—but chewing each bite one hundred times is ludicrous.

If chewing really isn't your thing, maybe brushing is. It's simply called the BRUSH-YOUR-TEETH DIET, and a lot of people do use this method to control their eating. I even read about several movie stars who do it—they're probably the ones who have contracts for toothpaste advertisements.

"I found that when I get the urge to eat and don't want to give in, I run to the bathroom and brush my teeth real fast. My mouth feels so fresh that I can't bear to destroy that feeling with food."

Looking at this diet seriously, you have to admit that brushing frequently may be great for your teeth, but it doesn't do a thing for your body. Besides, when was the last time you noticed a person with malnutrition having a great smile?

The HIGH-FIBER DIET became very popular when Dr. David Reuben learned that people in Africa were so healthy that they went to the bathroom daily because all their foods had a high fiber content.

Fiber is made up of cellulose, a complex carbohydrate that is not found in animal by-products. When you eat foods high in fiber, they stimulate your intestines and everything seems to move along a lot quicker.

So just as Stillman advocates water to push the food out of the body and Atkins suggested fats, Reuben and friends suggest fibrous foods as the magic power to make you lose weight.

"I read a diet that told me to sprinkle bran all over everything you eat. I put it all over breakfast, lunch, and dinner and I had the worst stomach aches in the world. And lord, did I spend a lot of time in the bathroom!"

The NATURAL-FIBER DIET can be a bit rough on your insides, and the whole idea of all that bran leaves my mouth dry. Fiber is important to your diet, but too much is just too much. If you eat a lot of fresh fruits and green leafy vegetables, you too will have regular bathroom habits (like those little guys in Africa who started this whole thing).

If the idea of eating a lot of bran makes you sick, this next one you won't believe. It's called the REGURGITATION DIET. Need I say any more?

The last of these personalized, dingy ways of dropping weight is the superdiet for the superrich called the COCAINE DIET. Cocaine (from the coca leaf, and from which Novocain is derived) comes in rock or cube form, and you pound it into a very fine powder. Then, with a straw or a spoon, you inhale it through your nose, and it sort of numbs the whole idea of eating.

Although this addictive habit is illegal, clever containers can be bought so you can carry cocaine everywhere just in case you are tempted by something fattening. The good coke will cost you around $150 a day; you will lose weight if you snort enough of it—you may also lose your nose if you use too much of it.

BIG-BROTHER DIETS

If for some reason you just can't seem to stick to a diet on your own, get out the Yellow Pages and you'll find a multitude of organizations claiming they can help you lose weight and keep it off. Dieting is a big business, as we've all noted, and many of these organizations are national or international in scope, with branch offices in every major city in the country, perhaps the world. (Except in India, where there are still plenty of starving children.)

These organizations are based on the thought that misery loves company and are usually headed by someone who has already taken off the weight and kept it off—naturally by the process now being taught at this diet center. Some are free, while others can cost you your weight in gold.

Jean Nidetch, a former chubby, began WEIGHT WATCHERS in 1963 in her living room, where she held meetings for her overweight friends so they could discuss their problems together. Her living room is now the world and franchises are located in every city you can think of, making it the largest international diet organization around. Weight Watchers has become so popular that Ms. Nidetch has spun off several cookbooks and a line of foods, including soft drinks, frozen dinners, and local ice cream.

It costs money to register and to attend each meeting.

"They make you take off your shoes, and they weigh you in every week and you sit in this room listening to people talk about how they lost their weight. I don't like being in a room with so many overweight people. I feel very self-conscious and I get bored with other people's problems. And I hate the way their food tastes. I quit after a while, but I did lose some weight. I think the idea of having some friends who understand your problem and who are supportive is very important."

Ms. Nidetch has since sold Weight Watchers to a large corporation that plans to expand the entire operation. Who knows, soon you'll be able to walk into your favorite supermarket and buy Weight Watchers' low-cal shampoo for "thinner, healthier hair."

Second in popularity is OVEREATERS ANONYMOUS, a spinoff of Alcoholics Anonymous. These meetings are held anywhere from church basements to private homes and are free to all participants.

"For a couple of hours you sit through these sob stories and then they tell you to eat three moderate meals a day with nothing in between but a sugar-free soft drink. There are 101 books for you to buy that are supposed to help you through your weight loss, and also you are assigned an O.A. sponsor whom you can phone if you get hungry."

At Overeaters Anonymous they believe that overeating is a sickness that you will always have throughout your life. It cannot be cured but it can be arrested. They often bring religion into the meetings and ask for help from God. The devil, as we all know, is a piece of chocolate cake.

The idea of telling a person they have a disease (overeating is a disease?) that can only be controlled but never killed doesn't seem to be a positive way to help anyone lose weight. Even with God on your side, the terminal illness of fat is hard to cope with.

Next comes the SCHICK CENTER FOR WEIGHT CONTROL, currently located in California, Washington, Texas, and New York, with plans to expand everywhere. Their ad shows a celebrity, looking very trim and handsome, who tells you to call the Center so that your weight worries can be over.

The diet program is spread out over six months. Information, prices, and techniques are not discussed over the telephone should you call just to inquire; you must go in and chat for a while, and then take out your checkbook. And then you're in for a real shock, which is not the only shock you will get while at Schick.

The first shock is the price. The second shock is the way they get you to lose weight.

"You bring in foods that are your favorites, six of them. They take these foods in the back and I swear they doctor them up or do something to them before they bring them back out. Then you pick the food up, chew it, and it tastes awful. Then they make you spit it out. All the time you're doing all this you are hooked up to this machine that gives you a mild electrical shock during different phases of your eating. I told all my friends, but they refused to believe me. I never went back and they wouldn't refund my money. That place is the worst."

I personally am so frightened of electricity and all related wattage that I swallow hard before changing a light bulb. The sight of a "diet electric chair" would automatically swear me off of fattening foods for a long time.

Besides the organizations we have just discussed, there are hundreds of smaller regional or local groups that claim to do as good a job for their members as the bigger and fancier ones. For many, losing weight among others who have the same problem is a very comforting thought. That security may one day help you to go the weight-loss route alone, and that's also a very comforting thought.

THE HEALTH-ADDICT DIETS

As interest in foods, nutrition, and health expands to more and more households, diets begin to emerge taking advantage of the health-food crazes and the newfound interest in keeping fit. These diets always sound solid, sturdy, and logical—almost in direct opposition to ding-dong diets. But that doesn't mean they're any better for you than the Jell-O and cotton-ball diet!

The MEGAVITAMINS DIET is based on the principle that if a few vitamin pills are good for you, a lot of vitamin pills will be *better* for you. But the truth about vitamins is that too many can be dangerous and actually poison your body. There are no proven facts about vitamin pills, and it is not at all advisable to live on vitamin pills instead of food.

"The food grown today is so filled with chemicals and depleted of natural vitamins that I have to take my own. I nourish my body daily with 160 vitamins. I don't take them all at once, needless to say."

Although capsules of miracles are a very big business these days, there is no reason in the world why a person who eats healthy, well-balanced meals should be taking 160 pills. At the moment, anyone who feels the pill need can get them in supermarkets, drugstores, and even door-to-door or purchased through the mail. Vitamin pills are easily accessible now, but the Food and Drug Administration is trying to pass a bill that will make certain vitamins *prescription only*. So before taking excessive dosages of Vitamin E, K, and pantothenic acid, check with the nutritionist or salesman who sold you these "dolls." While the one-a-day vitamin you were taught to take as a kid won't hurt you, more than that may. Even though our food today may be lacking a little quality, it's still the best way for our body to receive vitamins.

The ZEN MACROBIOTIC DIET is supposedly inspired by the Buddhist religion and the belief that everything in life is either *yin* or *yang*, which is not a Chinese version of the Hardy Boys. Yin and yang are opposites, so if you get ill, you've lost the balance between the two, which is a no-no. The macrobiotic diet stresses proper balance for your body through eating brown rice, a minimal amount of vegetables and seaweed, and tea. Many doctors have found this so-called "healthy way of life" quite dangerous, with anemia and severe vitamin deficiencies as results.

Dr. Kempner, of the Duke University School of Medicine in North Carolina, borrowed a few yins and yangs from the Buddhists to come up with the FAMOUS RICE DIET, which has been successful for almost fifty years. You should not attempt this diet yourself; it must be supervised by a hospital or doctor. If you really don't like rice, scratch this one off your list.

Do you like vegetables? Good, maybe the VEGETARIAN DIET is right up your garden. Did you know that Leonardo da Vinci, Benjamin Franklin, and Einstein were vegetarians? I knew that would impress you!

There are many kinds of vegetarians. Some do not eat any animal foods (meat, fish, or fowl) at all, including foods that come from any animal source; others will drink milk and eat eggs and cheese.

Whether you become a vegist because you don't think it's right to kill animals, hate the taste of meat, or just want to follow Einstein's Theory of Celery is not important. The trick vegetarians have to learn is how to get protein for their bodies in the absence of meat products. Beans, grains, and nuts are the answer. If this plate of greens sounds good, give this way of living a try. It can't hurt. I mean look at the Jolly Green Giant.

The next step up on the health ladder, vegetarian or otherwise, is the ORGANIC-FOODS DIET. If you choose to lead a purer life, you must insist on purer vegetables and fruits grown on land fertilized with manure and mulch. If you eat meat, you need to make sure it comes from ranch cows fed only organically grown grains. Same for your poultry, etc. Forget about the so-called "synthetic and pumped full of chemicals" food found in the supermarkets. One thing you won't be able to forget about is the food bill, if you decide to go "natural."

After much investigation the federal government has found no evidence that organically grown foods are any better for you than the ones you buy in the grocery store. If it makes you feel any better knowing the carrots you are serving on your dining-room table saw sun in Oregon and cost twice as much, then you should have those carrots (just don't expect bionic eyes overnight).

As you become a pro in the health world, you are bound to hit upon one of the oldest (and cheapest) healing techniques known to man. FASTING was practiced in ancient times to give the body a rest and to cleanse it of impurities.

The Bible tells us of holy people who would wander around the olive trees praying and going on a complete fast for forty days (you've really got to be holy to last that long without putting anything in your mouth besides prayers). Things have changed since the days of the Old Testament: fasting is now being used as a quick weight-loss technique. Magazines are filled with distilled-water or juice fasts that guarantee fast, thin results.

What exactly can you expect when you go on a fast and don't know what you're doing? First of all your stomach begins to grumble a lot and make funny noises. Your mouth starts feeling like a scene out of "Lawrence of Arabia," including the camel's breath. You are likely to get depressed, feel tired, and eventually lose interest in sex (lose weight and your mate). Nausea, dizziness, and sleepless nights follow—soon your blood pressure drops, vision blurs, the brain stops functioning, you fall into a coma and—bye-bye. Oh, yes, it's true about the weight—you do lose it.

On the other hand, if you do know what you're doing and are supervised by a doctor or hospital, fasting a day or three results in a physiological rest for your insides. Studies have proven that when an individual fasts only to melt off pounds, the loss is usually not permanent. Experts seem to believe the transition from eating nothing to being allowed food again is what causes a weight regain. (Do not attempt a fast without doctor's approval.)

If any of these diets really worked, none of the others would have had to be invented, right? Of course right. And the fact that there are sooooo many different kinds of diets with sooooo many different gimmicks to them really makes you wonder about the whole process, doesn't it?

I personally think that dieting stinks. I've done it as much as you have—maybe more—and I know that you can't live a normal life on an abnormal diet. It'll make you crazy, and it might make you unwell. Dieting, in fact, is just another form of mistreating your body—just like eating the wrong amount of food or the wrong kind of food and at the wrong time of day.

If I think dieting is rotten, why am I writing another diet book? Aha—got ya there. Well, the whole reason this book is called the *Never-Say-Diet Book* is because I just don't believe in diets. Instead, I believe in:

- Exercise—and plenty of it
- The right Live-It Program for your body
- Proper mental attitude

Stick with me, sweetheart. This really is the last diet book you're ever going to read.

THE WHAT ARE YOU PUTTING IN YOUR MOUTH QUIZ (AFTER YOU'VE READ THIS CHAPTER)

Okay, now, you've read all about breakfast, lunch, dinner, snacks, and diets. But reading isn't going to reduce your hips very much. You have to practice what I preach. When faced with a food choice, you are the only one who can change your life. So take this quiz and see how you do in real food situations.

If you get more than three answers wrong (including the trick question) go back to the beginning. You must have been eating something naughty the last twenty pages or so instead of paying attention! You're the one who needs to lose weight, remember? I've already lost one hundred and twenty-three pounds, and I didn't do it while eating and reading.

1. You go to a birthday party where you are served cake and ice cream on the same plate. You decide to eat:

a. everything (who wants to be rude?).

b. just the ice cream or just the cake.

c. a taste of each and quit.

2. You want to keep in tip-top shape, so you start your morning off with:

a. 500 milligrams of vitamin C.

b. glass of freshly squeezed orange juice.

c. Hi-C fruit drink.

3. Walking along the streets of a quaint vacation village, you see several different food vendors selling goodies. You stop at the:

a. pastry shoppe.

b. cheese shoppe.

c. chocolate shoppe.

4. The recipe calls for raspberries, which are currently out of season. You choose instead:

a. something else in season.

b. canned raspberries.

c. frozen raspberries.

5. The movie climaxes as the three-eyed cyclops from the deep is about to eat Cincinnati. You can't take a second more of suspense without a visit to the snack bar. You choose:

a. a hot dog and mustard with onions.

b. popcorn.

c. chocolate-covered yogurt bon-bons.

6. For tonight's special salad, you need an appropriate dressing. At the market you choose:

a. the fancy kind in the refrigerator section of the store.

b. the bottled kind that says low-cal.

c. the ingredients for a homemade vinaigrette.

7. To your cup of coffee you add:

a. one teaspoon of sugar (raw, brown or good ol' white).

b. one pack of Sweet 'n Low.

c. one spoonful of honey.

8. In avoiding junk foods, you go to your local health-food store and stock up on one of these low-calorie, dietetic, home-grown treats:

a. fruit and nut mix.

b. health carob bar.

c. soft yogurt with topping.

9. At a monthly luncheon for business people in your field, a pre-ordered meal of chicken in cream and wine sauce, string beans dripping in butter and almonds, and wild rice is served. You eat:

a. a fruit plate you asked the waiter to get you.

b. the chicken without the sauce (good luck scraping it off).

c. just the string beans.

10. You must have a piece of bread or cracker from the basket on the table or faint. Your choice is:

a. a piece of Rye Crisp.

b. a sourdough roll.

c. the heel of a piece of raisin pumpernickel rye.

ANSWERS

1. It's not fair to count on you to pass up completely the cake and ice cream, so, failing that, eat a few bites of each, put down your fork, and blow up a couple of balloons.

2. The fresh-squeezed orange juice is by far the best choice. Even a fresh orange is preferred over the other two choices.

3. You shouldn't even be sniffing the air around the pastry and chocolate shops. While some cheeses are fattening, they are not as bad for you as the sweet things. Try to find a skim-milk cheese, and enjoy.

4. Fresh is always going to be the correct answer (you should know that by now). After that, frozen or canned (no sugar) as a final desperate choice. It pays to reconsider any recipe that calls for canned goods.

5. Unsalted, unbuttered popcorn is the only choice. If it comes presalted and buttered, just go back to the monster and hope he eats you, too. When you get home, if it's not too late you can fix yourself some fresh popcorn (or next time pop some at home and take it with you to the movies).

6. Dressings in the refrigerator department are more expensive because they have extra mayonnaise or sour cream and fancy labels. So-called "low cal" dressings on the shelves are loaded with synthetics and poisons. Go home, mix up a little oil, some wine vinegar, some garlic, some Dijon mustard, and enjoy yourself.

7. I would never recommend the Sweet 'n Low, no matter how few calories it has, because it contains just too many synthetics and chemicals we know too little about. The honey is a bit more fattening, but it's better for you than any of the sugars and it gives your coffee a special zing.

8. There are no correct answers to this question (ha, ha, got you on this one). Anything you need in a health-food store can also be bought—for less money—in a grocery store. Go to you local A&P and get the yogurt (you don't need the topping). The health carob bars are very similar to candy bars, and the fruit and nut mix (a good idea for a snack, if you limit the amount) is cheaper at the grocery and not as good for you as fresh fruit.

9. Boy, you learn quick! Good for you. It's the fruit salad, of course.

10. Although bread is usually a no-no while you're weight conscious, you'll be happier (and so will your body) with a cracker. Start shopping around for crispy thin breads and wafers. Chewing them is good exercise for your teeth.

EXERCISE AND
THE LIVE-IT PROGRAM

INTRODUCTION

My parents always preached the benefits of exercise. A day didn't go by that someone in the house (including our 250-pound housekeeper, Berta) didn't give me a sales pitch on the importance of exercise.

Yet I can't recall one time that I ever saw my parents participating in anything that even slightly resembled exercise. I mean, if huffing and puffing was so wonderful and important why weren't Mom and Dad out on the lawn doing jumping jacks and cartwheels? Why were they so worried about making sure I didn't miss a tumbling class or a tap lesson, but so careless when it came to their own well-being?

The truth, though it's painful to admit, is that they didn't love themselves enough to give their bodies maximum care. They never believed anything could or would happen to them. They thought they were immortal, that the heart attack, the clogged arteries, the stroke, and the diseases only happened to someone else. They did not practice what they preached about exercise because they were not fully educated to the real facts of life. And believe me, when you find out that your own parents don't know the facts of life, it is a big shock!

I took my first formal, legitimate exercise class from a woman who was certainly an army sergeant at a boot camp in her previous life: I was screamed at, pulled on, and beaten into submission while the word *no* kept seeping through my screaming lips. Although I hate to admit this, I had to be driven home from the class by a friend because my entire body went on strike and didn't talk to me for three days.

After that experience, if anyone mentioned the word exercise to me, my thighs began shaking.

So now you must be asking yourself why the hell I picked this career, knowing full well that my body is allergic to any sort of physical exertion. I asked myself the same question every time I went back to exercise class.

And then, one day I didn't have to ask any more. I saw that my body—for the first time, I might add—looked really good. I felt so alive and powerful that I knew right then and there that I never wanted to look any different ever again. I never wanted to return to my previous shape. I never wanted to be in fat commercials again. I never, ever wanted to be an ugly duckling again.

It wasn't hard to figure out that if I truly wanted to be a swan, I would have to continue exercising regularly.

THE EXERCISE LIFE-STYLE TRUTH-OR-CONSEQUENCES QUIZ

Okay, okay, I caught you—thumbing through this chapter, wondering if you can skip it, looking ahead to the pretty pictures and the fancy photography, trying to wriggle your way out of the lecture. Well, it won't work.

Exercise is going to be your salvation—so if you don't want to be saved, well, that's another story. Otherwise, get your fat hands out of the other sections of the book and take this baby one page at a time.

You see, before we really get into exercise you have to take this little exercise quiz. It should be most helpful because it'll show you exactly where your insides stand compared to your outsides—and that may be something you don't happen to know right now. There's also the fact that a lot of people really sincerely believe that they get enough exercise when all they do is walk briskly through the frozen-food department of their local supermarket twice a week and circle the better-dress department on Saturday mornings. But because these people *think* they are getting enough exercise, they regularly ignore the thought of doing anything which may raise a little perspiration.

So here we go with another quiz. Throw away that skinny little pencil you've been clutching and pick up a nice heavy pen to jot down your answers. And no erasing!

1. As of today, do you participate in a regular exercise program?

   a. yes.

   b. whenever I have time.

   c. no.

2. Given a choice of climbing a few flights of stairs or taking the elevator, do you:

   a. always take the stairs?

   b. only take the stairs when the elevator is broken (complaining about Mr. Otis and his damn contraption all the way up the stairs)?

   c. always take the elevator?

3. When it comes to sports (football, basketball, skiing, tennis, etc.), do you:

a. fit sports into your weekly schedule on a regular basis?

b. get involved in sports on weekends, certain seasons, or every now and then?

c. only watch TV?

4. If you are sitting comfortable in your favorite Morris chair (what kind of chair is a Morris chair?) and need something in another room, do you:

a. get up and get it?

b. call for someone to bring it to you?

c. forget about it?

5. When you have to go to the store located a few blocks from your home or office, do you:

a. walk to the store?

b. drive to the store?

c. ask if they deliver?

6. After eating a big meal, do you:

a. walk around the block a few times?

b. promise to walk around the block a few times tomorrow?

c. get sleepy, and walk into the bedroom, and lie down like a dead tuna?

7. When the alarm rings in the morning, do you:

a. get out of bed and head for the bathroom?

b. crawl out of bed and try to make it to the bathroom?

c. check the time and roll over for a cat nap?

8. When you lie down to go to sleep, do you

a. go to sleep immediately?

b. toss and turn a bit before falling asleep?

c. need medication to relax you so you can sleep?

9. When someone asks you to join him or her in a physical activity (other than sex), do you:

a. join in if you can?

b. join in if you're in the mood?

c. say, "No thanks, that hurts my back," and continue reading the *Wall Street Journal?*

10. Which do you consider exercise:

a. bending, stretching, yoga?

b. swimming, jogging, tennis, football?

c. housework, gardening, cooking?

How to score:
All (a) answers are worth 2 points
All (b) answers are worth 3 points
All (c) answers are worth 4 points

_____ *20–24 POINTS* _____

YOU'RE DOING FINE: You are active, cheerful, and careful to take care of your body. You know when to get up and move around and you probably know how best to exercise your body for your own life-style. Your bathroom habits are regular and your skin is clear, but you can still do better.

_____ *25–29 POINTS* _____

ONLY HALF OF YOU SEEMS TO BE WORKING:

And don't ask me which half. It's a miracle you have the strength to pick up this book. You get tired in the afternoon, work too long and too hard in the office without enough time off for yourself, and have no idea of what you should be doing to take better care of your body. You are a walking time bomb. You're fine today. Five years from now you won't be.

30–40 POINTS

HOW DO I BREAK IT TO YOU GENTLY? You're in a lot of trouble and you're headed for a lot of unpleasant detours in life. You're a bit spoiled, awfully lazy, and even rather unimaginative. You get colds easily and spend way too much money at the drugstore on cure-alls that never work. Your idea of exercise is the walk from the parking lot to your office building each morning. You'd better start memorizing this book if you plan on living much longer.

WHAT'S YOUR EXCUSE?

I've tried a bunch of exercise programs and haven't come across one that holds my interest. I love Monopoly, card games, and Boggle, but I guess they don't count.
—The Weight Papers

The general consensus is that exercise is a real drag and not entertaining in the least. Entertaining, do you love it? You want maybe the Academy Awards? I can understand completely that many people look upon exercise as a drudge. But I happen to think that big hips, roly-poly thighs, tremendous calves, gigantic waistline tires, and flabby upper arms are also a drudge.

As for boring—anything can be boring. Even your own company. And you know

where boredom leads you—right to the refrigerator door. You'll do a lot better to be bored in an exercise class than out of it. And besides, you might like it better after a while.

"A friend of mine who exercises all the time told me that I was not really bored with the idea of exercising, that I was really afraid of succeeding and that's what turns me off to exercise, and I think he's right."

Not exercising may be a good excuse for how you got a Moby Dick complex, but it's still just an excuse.

Exercising around people is the trick. It's more challenging, more fun (remember, misery loves company), and more supportive.

"I called up a friend once and asked her if she would come to the gym with me because I didn't want to go alone. She called another friend who called someone else and that's how the whole thing got started. Three days a week, nine of us met after work and we had a ball exercising together. I tell you exercise has become such an important part of my life now, it gets boring on the nights off."

"I'd love to exercise, but I can't. I'm just too busy." This old standby excuse pops up any time you don't want to do anything. Have you ever met anyone too busy to watch the Super Bowl? Or a rerun of "Casablanca" on the afternoon movie? Of course not. You're never too busy to do what you want to do. And because you don't want to exercise, well, you'd come up with any old excuse.

People who use the too busy excuse usually back up their decision with reasons that are supposed to make it "all right." This method of rationalizing convinces them that they are getting the proper exercise as part of their busy day.

"I walk my German shepherd dog a few times a day and I spend several hours doing housework. I have a car pool on Mondays and Fridays. I cook the meals, clean the house, run the errands. You tell me when I'm going to have time for an exercise program. Besides, I do so much running around that it's equal to the exercise I'd get in a class."

Wrong. Unless you are a professional athlete or a gym teacher, the work you do to make a living is not giving you enough exercise for you to be able to forget this chapter of the book.

What you need to realize is:

1. You have to make time for the important things in life, and exercise is one of those things.
2. Exercise can make your busy day even more productive.

It's all a matter of organization. If you juggle your day properly, I guarantee you there are fifteen minutes at the same time of each day that you could be exercising, and there may be more.

Make up a schedule of your time so you can get a good look at how you're programming your day. List your basic activities, duties or roles in this space:

Wake up

_____

Eat breakfast

_____

_____

_____

_____

Eat lunch

_____

_____

_____

_____

_____

Eat dinner

_____

_____

Go to sleep

Now compare your list with this one I have made up for you based on a twenty-four-hour day:

Sleep	8 hours
Eat (one hour per meal)	3 hours
Rise-and-shine time in the morning	1 hour
Work	8 hours
Transportation to and from work	1 hour
Miscellaneous (writing letters, going to funerals, visiting dentist, watching TV, etc.)	2 hours

The total is twenty-three hours. You have one hour a day in which to exercise. Believe me, if you exercised one hour a day, you'd look terrific! And you'd feel better, too.

If that hour gets lost somehow, you can cut fifteen minutes from your telephone conversation to save your life. You can get up fifteen minutes earlier to prolong your life by ten years. Can you make time to save time? Of course you can.

When I was a kid, I never had to participate in P.E. class. I had a running (actually mine was limping) list of doctor's excuses to prevent me from making a fool out of myself: asthma, hay fever, sinus attacks, flat feet, and of course, a very serious weight problem. So while everyone else was huffing and puffing away in their little blue shorts and white shirts, I was reading *Valley of the Dolls* and finishing off a box of Nabisco Vanilla Wafers.

Everyone has been sick at one time or another. But there are several different categories of sick when it comes to excusing oneself from exercise. I think you have to be sick not to exercise, so let's take a look at a few of these categories and see if you've ever been guilty of these low crimes.

Each of the categories has a line after it, you will note. With a pencil—don't use pen, you'll be embarrassed later and you won't be able to erase—make a check mark if you've ever been in that specific category. Ready?

Make-Believe Illnesses_____

Inventing aches and pains is extremely easy to do. You can come up with all kinds of sicknesses in just a few minutes' time and just about everyone will believe your tale of woe. Pretty soon you'll even believe it yourself.

"My friends tell me I'm an imaginary invalid. I continue to bring about these moments of physical anguish over and over again." There are psychosomatic illnesses in which you really do develop the illness, but the reasons are psychological rather than pathological ones, and there are plain old fakers who are sick whenever they want to get out of doing something they consider unpleasant. While make-believe illnesses may prevent you from exercising, they haven't prevented you from eating, and there is nothing imaginary about the extra pounds lying around your middle.

Temporarily Out of Order_____

You weren't eating right—you didn't get enough sleep—you've been working too hard, and now you're in bed with the flu, a stomachache, a headache, or *la grippe*. Your strength is gone and it's best to stay in bed for repairs. Naturally you swear on a stack of Tylenol tablets that as soon as you're feeling better you'll be back at exercise class. Once you recover you'll start jogging again. Once you're back in shape things will be different. Or so you say.

Ten days later you still haven't gotten into the swing of things. "Maybe tomorrow I'll exercise." And maybe tomorrow you'll be temporarily sick again.

Setback by Nature_____

This is a very special category which concerns people with physical limitations. Unfortunately, we aren't all created physically equal. Sometimes Mother Nature makes a mistake or two and some people come out different than others. As unfortunate as it is, it's a part of reality that cannot be ignored.

Physically handicapped people can and should exercise. In fact, if their handicap has specific confinements, they may need to exercise even more than nonhandicapped people. As rights and realities of the handicapped become a political issue, more and more exercise programs geared to the handicapped will open up. If you don't know of a program in your neighborhood, put one together with your friends. You don't have to be able to perform a perfect jumping jack to appreciate exercise.

"I always felt sorry for myself and had a lot of hate in my heart for everyone because of my own misfortune. When things got really tough for me I joined a handicapped program at a free clinic near my home. I cannot begin to tell you what a difference it has made in my life. Not only have I begun to accept so many things I wouldn't face for so long, but now I have the confidence mentally and physically to go out there in the world and make it."

Side Effects

The world is made up of a lot of clumsy, klutzy people who don't pay attention to what they are doing. By accident, or almost on purpose, they fall out of buildings, get hit by moving vehicles, and suffer the meanest of slings and arrows. They end up going through a lot of pain and undoubtedly wind up on medication, in therapy (physical or mental), and stuck with a long rest-and-recuperation period.

After the accident and the recuperation, many people are afraid to attempt any kind of extra exercise, thinking it will hurt too much or they will undo the mending arts of Mother Nature. This is a big mistake. If you fall off a horse, you know you've got to get back up there and ride that devil. If you lose some movement in your body temporarily, you've got to get back in there and exercise it to work out the kinks of disuse.

If your accident has left you with immobile parts for any extended period of time, you're going to have to exercise those parts slowly to bring them up to optimum condi-

tion. Even learning how to walk again is a matter of exercise. It should be taken slowly and carefully—often with professional help. But you must return to exercise if you want to return to your former self.

And while you're recuperating—ask your doctor if there are any exercises you can do to keep in shape or help chase the pounds away while you are whiling away time.

I'm Pregnant

Many pregnant women are afraid to exercise. They're afraid they'll hurt themselves, their unborn babies, or just exhaust themselves during a time when they're already tired.

These are mostly misconceptions—yuk yuk. Sure there are pregnancies that are more difficult than others. There are even pregnancies when you have to stay in bed for months. But many doctors applaud exercise for pregnant women, especially for women who have been exercising regularly prior to conception.

NEVER BEGIN AN EXERCISE PROGRAM DURING PREGNANCY WITHOUT YOUR DOCTOR'S APPROVAL. If you are already in good shape through exercise, there will probably be no objections from your doctor. I've exercised women up to the end of their eighth month of pregnancy—and even later.

Cher exercised until the week before her son Elijah was born.

"During my first pregnancy I was scared to do anything that would shock or upset the baby. I wanted to do everything right, so I really took it easy. I've got to tell you I had no strength anyway. The next time I got pregnant I kept up my exercise classes and it made a world of difference. I think it was good not only for me but for the baby as well."

There are many advantages to staying in shape during pregnancy:

◇ ◇ ◇

1. Exercise improves circulation. It's important to keep all systems going in order to give your coming attraction optimum health. Exercise helps keep the juices flowing.

2. Exercise aids posture. Carrying a baby is a strain on the back, neck, shoulders, and legs. You can give yourself extra strength in these areas through exercise.

3. Exercise relaxes you. There are many tense moments during pregnancy, and it's important to release those tensions so they don't stay inside you. A relaxed mother is a healthy mother, with a healthy baby.

4. Exercise keeps water weight down. NEVER EXERCISE DURING PREGNANCY WITHOUT YOUR DOCTOR'S CONSENT. (I'm really serious about that, or I wouldn't have said it twice.)

EXERCISE FALLACIES

Many people don't like to exercise because they think it will actually harm them. They suffer from lack of information. Proper exercise will harm very few people. Let's examine some of the common myths and fallacies and see if we can end your fears:

"... *I'm Too Heavy*. I have to lose weight before I can exercise regularly." Bullshit. Sure, if you resemble the American buffalo you have a reason to worry about falling over dead after a six-mile jog. But even buffaloes can begin an exercise program slowly and work up to more strenuous activity as their bodies adjust.

I don't suggest sky diving, wrestling in Madison Square Garden (or out of it), or marathon mountain climbs when you aren't in the peak of physical condition.

In fact, the heavier you are the lighter your exercises should be. The more excess baggage you are carrying on you, the more careful you have to be. But this doesn't mean you shouldn't exercise at all. It simply means you must go slowly on a supervised (by an M.D.) plan. Diet and exercise should be combined, and the exercise will actually help you in your first attempts to make a dent in your figure.

"... *I'm afraid my fat will turn to muscle*." Fat is fat and muscle is muscle. Got that? Fat cannot turn to muscle, and vice versa. If you exercise but continue to eat like a horse, you will never lose weight. In fact, the fat surrounding your muscles will just become firm and solid, and before you know it, you'll look—and feel—like a Brink's truck.

If you are careful about the food you put in your mouth and continue your regular exercise program, you will lose weight. Exercise will break up the fat while it tones and works the muscles of the body. Exercise will not turn your fat into muscle. Besides, you should be a lot more worried about a dead body than a muscular one.

"... *Exercise makes me hungry*." Television ads can make you leap across the room to stuff your face. Watching other people eat can start your mouth watering. Smelling fresh-baked bread can make you desperate for a few slices. But you have hit rock bottom if you believe that exercise can make you hungry.

Many things can make you hungry. Many others may arouse your appetite. Exercise can do neither. There is a very big difference between appetite and hunger. Hunger is very real. Your body calls out for fuel to keep it going. Appetite feels like hunger, and you'd swear it was real, but it is purely psychological. That's why you get "hungry" when you're bored, lonely, depressed, or whatever.

If you have an appetite after exercising, it is a psychological problem and not a physiological one. Honest.

If during exercise you are thinking of a cold meatball sandwich with potato salad, a sour pickle, and a Pepsi, you certainly will be hungry when you finish up your one-two-three-fours. But if you concentrate on your exercises and your body tone, you will not be hungry after the session. Many people, in fact, say that exercise helps control their appetite.

"After I finish working out I feel so healthy and alive. I make an effort not to eat very much after I exercise. I mean, I just burned off some fat and calories and I'm not in a hurry to put them back on. I feel so exhilarated that I want to go out and conquer the world, not a restaurant. I might be thirsty after exercise, but never hungry."

". . . I'm too old, exercise wouldn't help." If you think about growing old and ending up in "Pleasant Acres" making baskets and molding clay, you will certainly fulfill your own prophecy of doom. If you refuse to accept the idea of aging, chances are you will outlive all your friends.

You always hear about the little old lady who at the age of eighty-six runs several miles and goes mountain climbing with her grandchildren. I'm not telling you to take her as a role model. I mean, that's great for her, but I don't think it's the only way to go! You merely owe it to yourself to exercise regularly and keep in shape.

"Those who say they don't believe exercise helps us old folks have lost their marbles. I would have gone senile without it. Everyone tells me how wonderful I look for my age. Well, I owe it all to exercise. Keeping fit keeps me out of the obituary columns. You can bet on it."

Every now and then I visit a retirement home and teach a very mild exercise class. You cannot believe the excitement, renewed energy, and lift in morale generated from that twenty-minute class. You don't have to send your grandmother out to a disco every night, but make sure she gets up out of that rocking chair—and fast!!!

ARE YOU GETTING ENOUGH?

There are a lot of different theories in this world about exercise. Obviously there wouldn't be so many books, so many fancy store fashions, or so many businesses based on slimming and trimming if there weren't room for a lot of discussion.

So, needless to say, I have my own theory. I believe that there are many forms of exercise that are excellent for you, your figure, and your insides. If you jog, play tennis, or do aerobic dancing, I think that's great. But when you are combining a weight-loss program with an exercise program, I happen to believe that you need a serious series of exercises to enhance your total being rather than a swift game of ball chasing on a clay court.

Now don't get me wrong. I'm not saying you can't play any more tennis on my program, that tennis is bad for you, or that you should give up any of your favorite activities. I'm simply saying that to lose the weight you need to lose and to keep it off, you must combine *my* exercise program with *my* food program or you won't get the results I'm promising you you deserve.

You can still play tennis, jog, or climb Mt. Everest. But there're no substitutions in this program. You *must* also do the exercises I prescribe for you later in this chapter.

I Walk, Jog, and Run—Why Should I Do More Exercises?

Some people believe that walking (leading up to running an eight-mile marathon) is the best kind of exercise and the most helpful way to take care of your heart. I do agree that walking steps up your circulation, which eventually strengthens and cleans out that red muscle beating on your left side. I don't agree about it being the *best* exercise around. So you have a better heart after knocking your brains out and leaping over puddles and poodle stools. So what? Do you think when you walk into a room people say, "Hey, look at Helen's heart. Isn't it terrific-looking? Wow, I'd like to take her heart dancing some time soon."

Unfortunately, walking and related strides don't do a great deal for many other body areas that need alteration. Too often, an overweighter will jump into a jogging suit and a groovy pair of running shoes and try to keep up with a six foot two inch basketball player who's been pounding the track for years. The hips, the double chins, the saggy arms don't benefit from all that huffing and puffing, and you're likely to suffer from knee problems, swollen Achilles' tendons, and heel pains along the way.

If you are into any of the above movements, fine, but don't kid yourself about walking your way to an hourglass figure. You have to walk fifteen hours to burn off one pound of fat—and the chocolate bar that takes five minutes (or less) to eat takes about an hour's worth of walking to burn off.

Rating:
Walking, running, jogging are partial exercises, not complete ones. If you have twenty pounds to lose I'd hate to be the one who pays for your shoes.

I Play a Lot of Sports . . .

First of all, what is a lot? Do you play tennis three or four times a week? How about racquetball, golf, horseback riding, and swimming? Do you fit any of these sports in your hectic weekly schedule? I'm not referring to the time you played softball on July Fourth or when you went bowling because a couple of friends asked you to join them one night. They don't count. If you're getting on a pair of skates or swinging a club just to be social, that's wonderful, but not enough.

Sports are sports and exercises are exercises. They are not exactly the same thing. All sports involve some degree of effort (exercise), but there isn't any individual sport that includes all the exercises your body needs to function correctly. Some people who play golf religiously still have a flabby fanny. Why? Because golf does nothing to tone and exercise that part of the anatomy. I have a friend who swims the way Esther Williams used to and has arms and legs like Ben Hai's. Why? Because swimming builds muscles and you can get stuck with unwanted and unattractive areas.

Rating:
If you are into the sports scene I'm all for it. Just make sure, though, you consider your whole body instead of perfecting only your backhand.

I Belong to a Health Club . . ._____

Belonging to a health club is like belonging to anything else you have a membership card to—if you don't use it, forget it.

You pay three hundred to six hundred dollars a year (plus a monthly fee) to obtain membership in a figure salon or body shop. Do you honestly make use of this luxury? How often? I'm not talking about going at your leisure to sit in the sauna, lie on the rooftop to sun, or meet a few friends for lunch. I'm talking about spending an hour or so at least three times a week and working that body of yours. It's not enough just to belong to one of these places, you have to make use of the professional help it offers, or it's no good.

If you have not yet joined a club and are considering it, be careful. Some are ripoffs, while others are legitimate operations that care. Before signing on the dotted line and handing over a check, check out the place and see that it's more than six sun lamps, a TV room, one small jacuzzi, and a stack of towels.

Rating:
Health clubs and the like can guarantee you to a membership of feeling and looking better forever. That's only if you go regularly. If not, this will just be more money you wasted on the fat cause.

I Exercise at Home with My Own Equipment . . ._____

Oh my, now we're getting very fancy. Who needs to go to a health club when you have all the devices right there in the comforts of your abode? Let me guess—do you have an exercycle? I bet you do.

Do you have the real professional one that tells you how many miles you go and the rate at which your heart is beating? Aren't those things marvelous, and so attractive sitting there in your dining room?

Maybe you own one of these mini trampolines that you have right by the bed, so you can spring out from between the sheets and jump around a few hundred times or so.

What about a tummy belt for wear around the middle area while you're gardening or doing housework? Does all that chrome and plastic apparatus just sit there like your membership card? Sorry to hear that. Dust is not good for overweight people, you know.

Every year the Federal Trade Commission seizes many of these advertised "wonder machines" and "reducing gadgets," referring to them as useless and dangerous. Some of the machines that are advertised each year (especially around bikini season) do pump your muscles up or strengthen your body, but there's not one that "melts away fat," believe me.

Rating:
The best equipment you have is your own body. All the springs, coils, and weights needed to exercise with are located somewhere between your head and your feet. Remember, you are the machine—you don't need another one that plugs into the wall to help you. You can do it by yourself.

I Go for Weekly Treatments for My Body . . .

The newest trend that is loosely defined as an exercise is the various massage techniques offered to those who believe that fancy rubdowns can rub out fat.

European experts have left their homeland to open up small salons all over America in order to share with us their slimming beauty secrets. The French are known for their romantic and suave approach to life—not so when you find yourself in a horizontal position and a pair of Parisian hands are about to give you a cellulite treatment. They knead, push, pull, and squeeze all your lumps of fat, but after all the pain you are as lumpy as ever.

The Swedes bake you in hot, dry saunas, then cool you in jacuzzis before showing you what Danish hands can do. (And all this time you thought Danish was soft gooey pastries.)

The ones you really have to be careful with are those ever smiling Oriental masseuses. Don't let all that tinkly music fool you: once you turn your back, they're right there walking on it.

The zenith of massage is called Rolfing, a series of very deep, painful tissue- and muscle-cleansing sessions. Many people swear Rolfing puts their whole body in alignment, and pounds seem to disappear. I went only once, and as this person began pressing hard on my eyeballs I surrendered (my eyeballs were the thinnest part of me).

There are as many different kinds of massages as there are masseurs. Some are soft, others hard, but none can rub away fat. You can get wrapped in cellophane or towels dipped in fancy herbs, and you will sweat off some water weight, but that's about all.

Rating:
Massages are wonderful—some tend to think they're better than sex! For relaxing purposes, a good rubdown cannot be beat. For losing weight, forget it.

EXERCISE VS. SPORTS

I've truly got nothing against sports—some of my best friends are sports—but I do insist that exercise is better for you when you're trying to take off weight.

It's always been amazing to me that people can be so quick with reasons why they can't exercise or lists of things that exercise doesn't do for them. I've never seen a list of what exercises *can* give you that nothing else can.

Exercise Helps Give You Self-Respect

Ego is essential for all of us to look and feel our best. If you want positive things to happen to you, you have to look and feel positive. Exercise builds up the ego because it is hard work that no one else can do for you—only you can conquer the exercises and only you can appreciate what you've done for yourself each day you succeed. Each day you do something positive for yourself and your body by exercising is a day when you can feel a little bit better about yourself for having made the effort. You begin to realize you can conquer anything.

Exercise Can Get You a Better Job

People who are unhappy with their appearance are usually frustrated. And frustrated people can be terrible workers. And we know what happens to terrible workers—they get fired. Or they never even get hired. And unemployed people are unhappy, so they eat, and when they eat they gain weight, and then . . . well, you know how the cycle works. You can protect yourself from this problem through exercise. We all know that the people who hire and fire are concerned about appearance and are already prejudiced in favor of thin people. Exercise that tones your body and improves your attitude and efficiency will not only help you keep your job but will make sure you're hired over someone else who may be equally qualified but is twenty pounds overweight.

Exercise Makes for Better Relationships

"I gave up trying to look like those fantastic people in the magazines and decided to do the best with what I had, and what I had nobody wanted. I joined a gym and met a lot of others who were in the same boat. But man, exercise really helped to make me a better me and that really showed. It gave me more self-confidence and that changed my appearance physically as well as mentally, and now I can relate much better because I'm not so defensive any more."

As I always tell my exercise students: you have to like yourself before you can expect anyone else to like you. In order to get to the point where you like yourself, you sometimes have to exercise your buns off. Once your mind and your body are on your side, you become a more stable and well-adjusted person, and then you are ready to find someone else to share your life with.

Exercise Improves Your Health

We all know this in general terms, so let's look at it very specifically:

1. Exercise can help correct posture, reduce fatigue, and increase efficiency.

2. Exercise keeps your mind working faster so you can avoid accidents better. You can also move more quickly to get out of the line of trouble.

3. Exercise controls blood pressure, which enhances your eyesight and hearing abilities. This also means you can drive better and get fewer tickets.

4. Exercise will give you stamina. You'll even be a better dancer.

5. Exercise will prime your body so that you require less sleep. You'll also feel more awake and alive when you are awake and alive. You won't walk around feeling drowsy or hung over when you aren't.

6. Exercise will improve your bathroom habits. It will also ease menstrual cramps.

7. Exercise will make your body heal more quickly. Even pimples will go away faster. Hair and fingernails will grow faster and stronger. Skin will take on a healthier glow.

8. Exercise will make sex better. "Sex is definitely a lot more enjoyable when you're in shape. I never had an orgasm in my life until I started taking care of my body." Need I say more?

9. Exercise can put money in your pocket. It's very simple. Because of exercise:

You like yourself better. THEREFORE: You can accomplish goals previously considered unreachable. THEREFORE: You are more secure, self-confident, relaxed, and creative. THEREFORE: You are worth more money.

EXERCISE THE LIVE-IT WAY

If you've tried the majority of diets and exercise programs we've discussed so far, and none of them has worked, you're probably wondering how I'm going to offer you something sensible that works.

Well, here it is.

The Live-It Program.

Take a look at the word diet. The first syllable is DIE, yes, DIE. Now is that any way to inspire anyone? So let's just take the word diet and junk it right now. Throw it out of your vocabulary and get rid of it now. Erase it from your memory bank.

Now replace diet with the word Live-It.

Yes, Live-It, because that's what you must be doing every day of your life. Living off a balanced, sensible food program, on a steady and life-giving exercise program, not for two weeks or two months, but forever.

My Live-It program breaks down into three equally important parts:

- The Live-It Exercise Program
- The Live-It Food Plan
- The Live-It Mental Exercises

Each is important to the success of the other—together the sum of the parts totals a new you. You will now begin to lose weight by exercising all your body, by cutting down your food intake, and by maintaining a healthy attitude, for a change.

WHAT CAN YOU EXPECT WHILE ON THE LIVE-IT PROGRAM?

We are all taught not to expect anything in life. If you do something nice for a friend and don't get a thank you or a few kind words you're supposed to smile and feel you did your good deed for the day. If you don't "expect," then anything positive that comes your way will be a nice surprise. In many cases that way of thinking is true; but in the Live-It Program you should have great expectations . . . and you will if you Live-It properly. I know your mind is just filled

with all the standard questions: "What can I expect, how fast will I see results, when will I be thinner?"

You've been persuaded time and time again that fat cells will just drop off your arms and legs and disappear on the carpet beneath you. There's this new package of diet pills out that boasts, "By the time this bottle is empty, you will be pounds thinner" (of course—you may be dead, and believe me you lose a lot of weight in the "thereafter").

But if you follow my food program, do your exercises and train that mind of yours to help you, you *will* see results. You shouldn't worry about how fast those results will take place. Every *body* is different. Metabolisms are different. You've been eating a certain way or not exercising for a long time. Your body will take time to adjust to all the changes, so don't be a time freak. Learn being a patient person.

Week one: The hardest of all because everything is new, different, and difficult. You may be cranky and tense. A bit sore from the exercise. You should also be proud that you've made it this far. If you can get through this week, you can make it to the end.

Week two: You're looser now and more comfortable. The results of exercise and breathing properly are beginning to show in your attitude. You will have lost three to six pounds by now.

Week three: You are settling into your new, good eating habits and seeing the benefits of your self-control. The weight is coming off and the exercise regime is actually beginning to feel good. Your attitude is improved and you are getting a high by seeing how far you've come.

Week four: You got it made! You've changed your life-style. You may consider cheating on eating habits or exercise, but a quick weight gain will show you what a bad idea this is. You are really on your way to a new you—permanently. Congratulations!!!

Weeks to come: You are continually learning about balance for your body. You have found out that you are able to eat a few of your all-time favorites and know you won't gain an ounce because you've also added a few more exercises to your weekly schedule. As your weight goes down and you start to firm up you may notice a few stretch marks on your body. No, they will not go away permanently. They are nature's way of reminding you what was and should never be again (don't forget a little body cream on those stretch marks, they love it!).

THE LIVE-IT EXERCISE PROGRAM

The Live-It Exercise Program is structured for all different body types and geared to help you lose weight no matter how much you weigh. Everyone, no matter how much he weighs, begins with a set of breathing exercises. After that, each person must find the proper program for his weight loss. There are three programs, depending on how much you need to lose. Thumb through the next few pages and find the category you fit into. Then, as you lose the necessary weight, move to the next category. If you have to lose more than fifty pounds, please consult a doctor before beginning this program.

Breathing Is Believing

Breathing and exercise go hand in hand, just like toast and jelly. (I really hated to use the comparison, but, well, I knew you'd understand.)

If you don't breathe, all body functions stop. You turn purple and die. Hello. Goodbye. Amen.

It's that simple. If you don't breathe properly (and 90 percent of you don't) then you are short-changing your body and depriving yourself of oxygen. And that could cause a multitude of problems.

Breathing, when done correctly, can be a great aid to losing weight because you will be getting rid of a lot of carbon dioxide. Carbon dioxide lives in all those cute little fat cells you're trying to get rid of and just helps them puff up and fill out.

At the beginning of each of my classes I tell my students, "I want to hear you breathe. I want to hear it real loud. You may get a little dizzy at first because the brain hasn't had that much good oxygen for a long time, but you'll get used to it soon.

"Blow it out," I shout, "blow it out."

Fat cells don't die, but they do get smaller and smaller, so before you begin any physical activity, you have to begin breathing properly.

You see, breathing sets everything in motion and cleans out the blood, revving up the old circulation and often giving you a natual high. Proper breathing can help calm you down during a crisis. Why, it even brings a healthier glow to your skin.

Sold? I knew you would be. So let's do a little breathing together.

1. First, blow your nose. We do not want a

mess all over the place—especially on the pages of this book.

2. Now take in some air through your nose. That's not exactly my idea of a good sniff. Try it again. Now take in some air and think about Mark Spitz.

3. Now blow it out through that mouth of yours. Blow it out. Blow it out.

THAT WAS PITIFUL!!!

I wish I were there to slap your lips. How do you expect that air to get inside your whole body when you are imitating a guppy in heat? I mean, really!

Now straighten up your back, stretch your neck, and let's try it again—and hold in your stomach.

1. Inhale through your nose (more! more! more!).

2. Okay. Hold it for the count of five:

ONE	THREE	FIVE
TWO	FOUR	

3. Now, very evenly, let out all that air while keeping your stomach tucked in and your back straight. Blow it out!

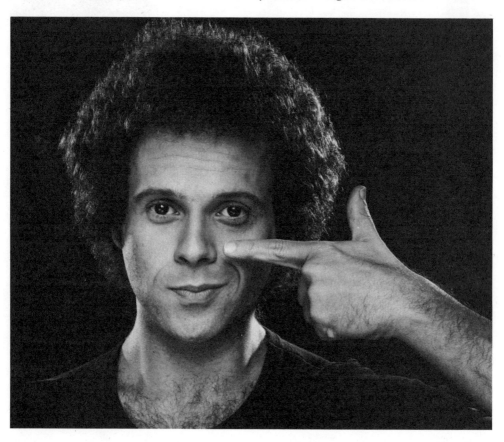

If you keep your stomach tucked in good and tight you get bonus points: it's like doing an exercise twice.

Now let's try this breathing stuff one more time. Breathing better is going to make a big difference in the way you feel and how you take off weight, so let's make sure you've got it down perfectly.

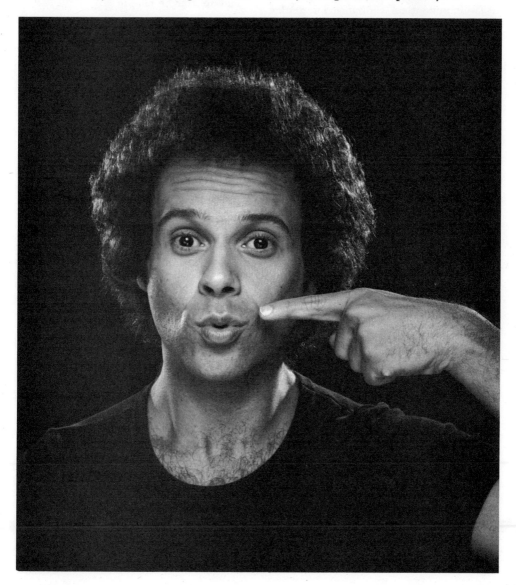

This exercise doesn't work as well, by the way, if you've got bad breath. So put the book down and go gargle with some mouthwash before we continue.

(Two-minute time allowance for getting breath fresh and clean.)

Good. You're back. I'm so glad. Here we go. Sit up straight, neck up, and:

1. Inhale through your nose (keep going, keep going, keep going, that's it!).

2. Keep that air in for the count of 100—just kidding. Hold for a count of five:

ONE	THREE	FIVE
TWO	FOUR	

3. Let out the air slowly, hold your stomach in, and relax. Good.

Now stand up. Keep your stomach in and stand up straight, chin in.

◇ ◇ ◇

1. Place your hands on your lower stomach—below the belly button.

2. Inhale a lot of air through your nose.

3. Slowly let the air out of your mouth and at the same time press gently on your tum. Keep pressing until you release as much air as possible. Blow it out. Let me hear you.

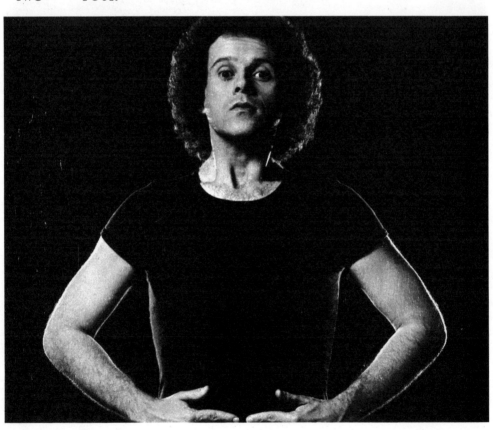

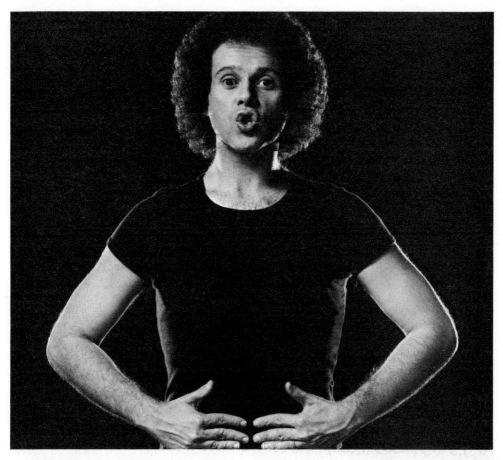

You shouldn't just breathe correctly when you are exercising. You must incorporate good breathing into all your activities:

DRIVING THE CAR
WALKING, JOGGING, OR RUNNING
PUSHING THE GROCERY CART
LYING IN BED
AT MEALTIMES
DURING SEX
AND WHENEVER ELSE YOU HAPPEN
TO BE BREATHING

Once you learn the techniques of expanding your lungs and letting the air out, sinus problems, emotional strain, and even headaches will be a thing of the past. So will big fat cells.

If you are *fifty pounds or over* I'm starting you off very slowly. But remember, as you lose the weight and fit into the next program, it's going to get tougher. But I know you can do it—just keep thinking positive and relax in the tub a little longer at night.

The First Five Minutes Every Morning

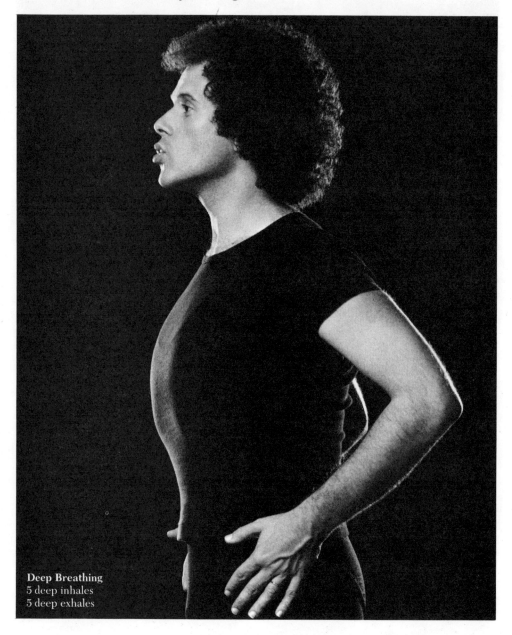

Deep Breathing
5 deep inhales
5 deep exhales

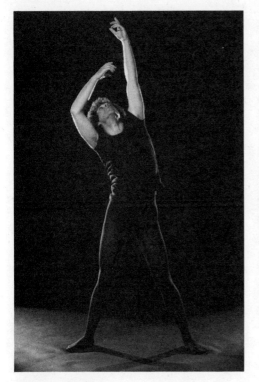 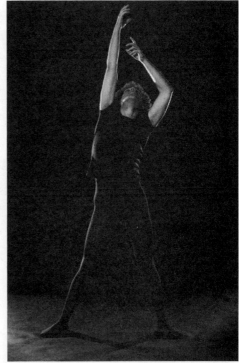

Climb and Stretch
20 climbs
10 with each hand

Side Bends
20 bends
10 to the left
10 to the right

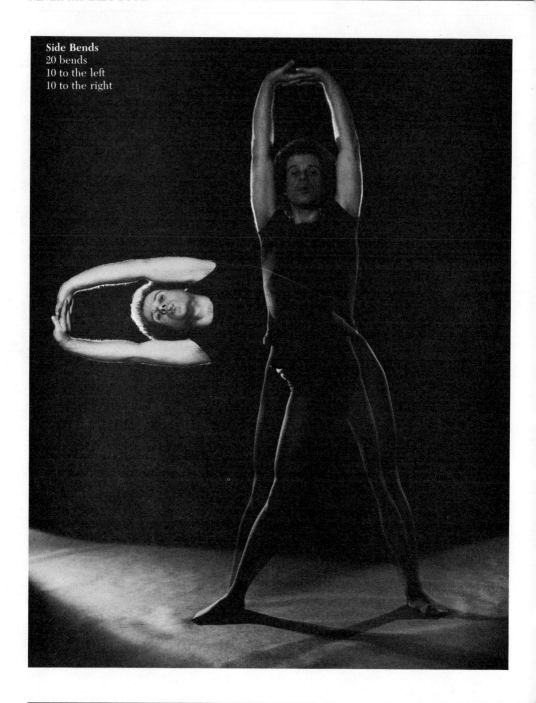

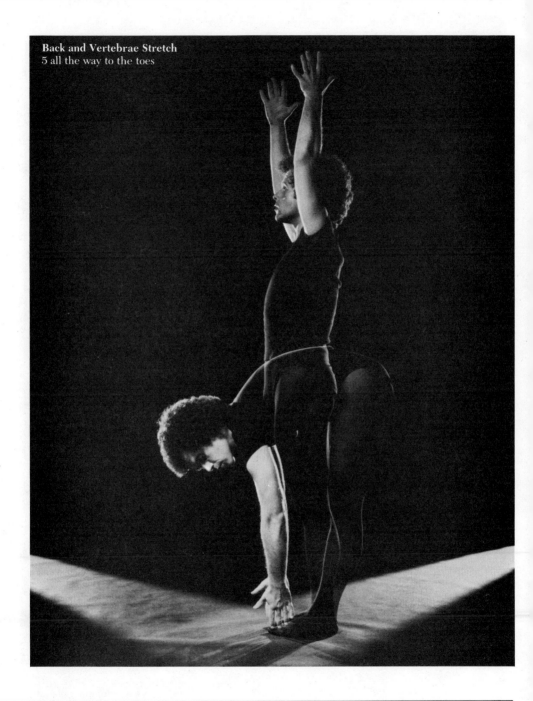

Back and Vertebrae Stretch
5 all the way to the toes

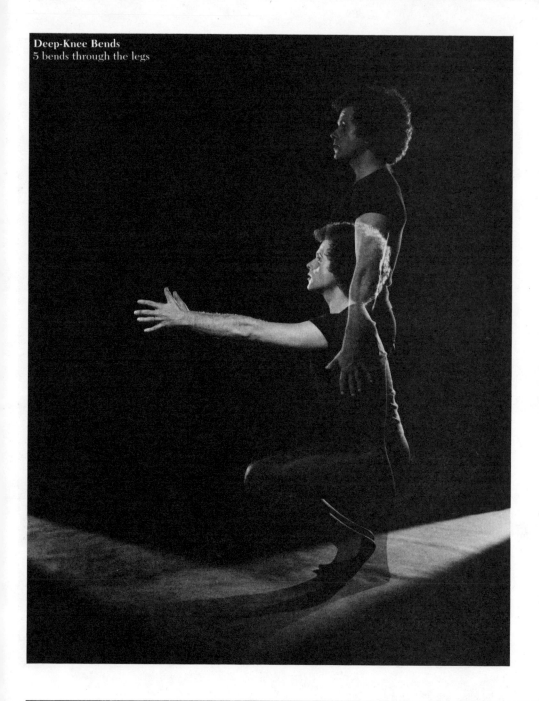

Deep-Knee Bends
5 bends through the legs

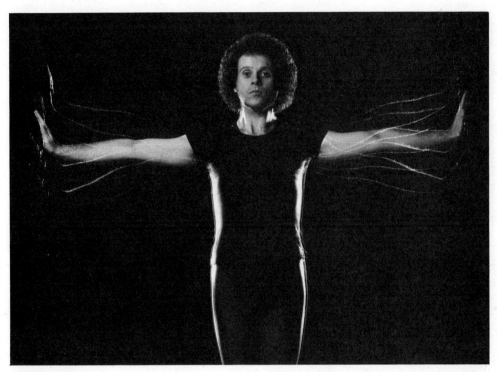

Arm Circles
10 clockwise
10 counterclockwise

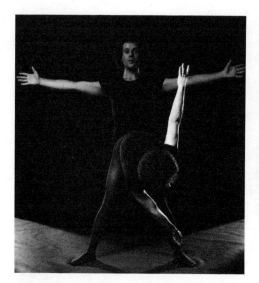 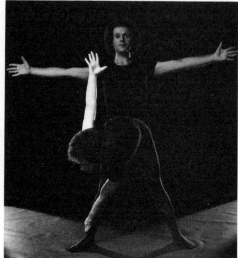

Toe to Toe
20 turns
10 to each foot

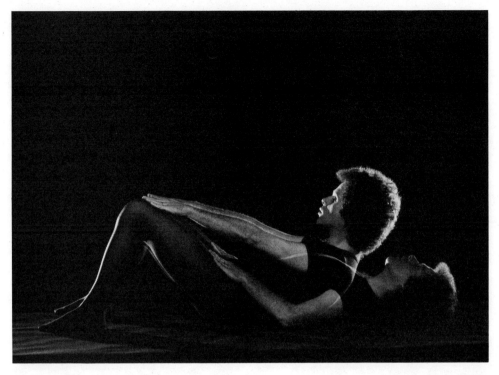

Mini Sit-ups
10

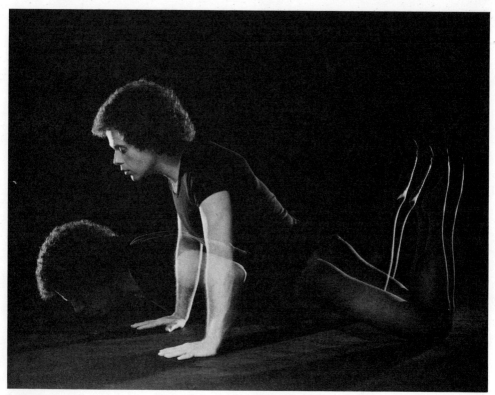

Mini Pushups
10

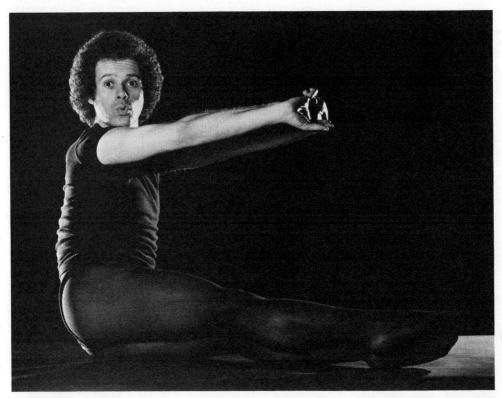

Tootsie Rolls
60
30 from cheek to cheek

*The Last Five Minutes in the Evening*___

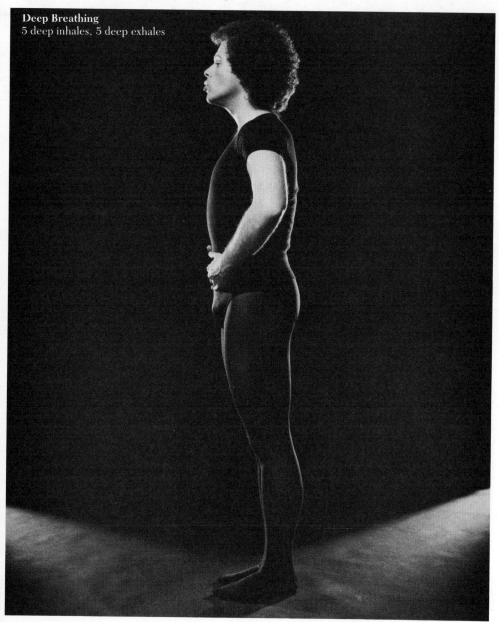

Deep Breathing
5 deep inhales, 5 deep exhales

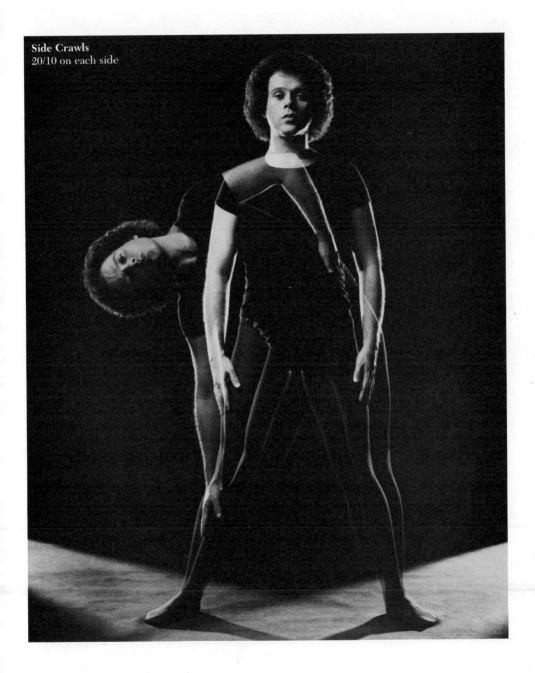

Side Crawls
20/10 on each side

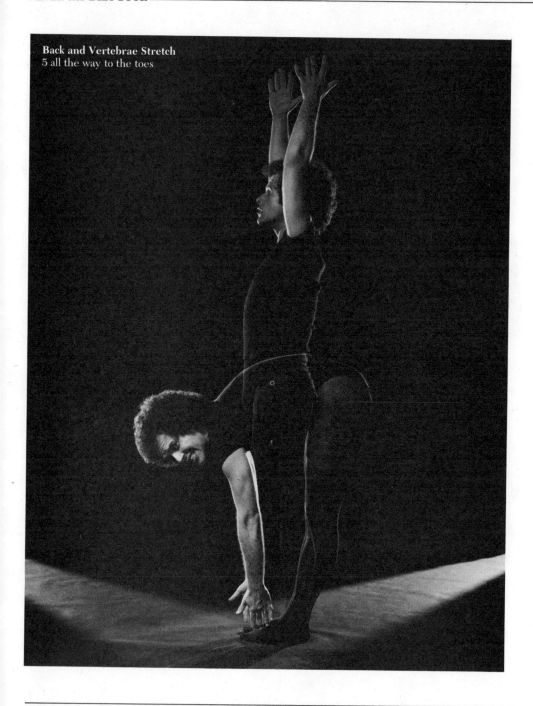

Back and Vertebrae Stretch
5 all the way to the toes

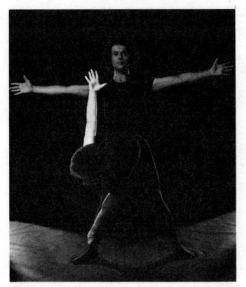 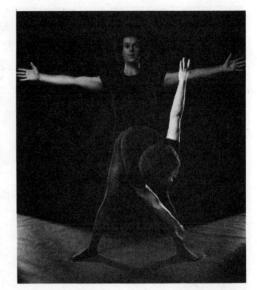

Toe to Toe
20 turns/10 to each foot

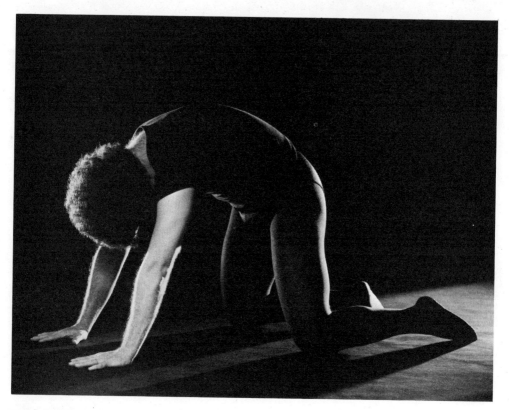

Cat Stretch
5 inhales, 5 exhales

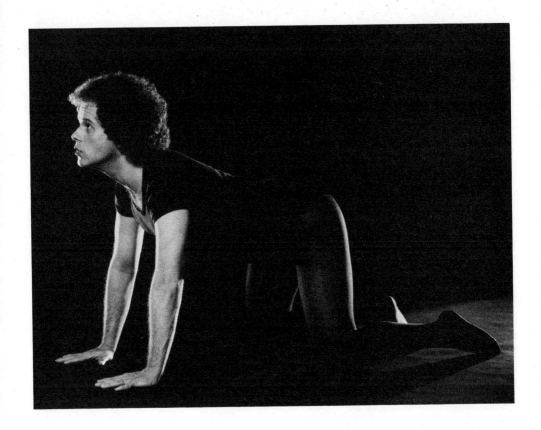

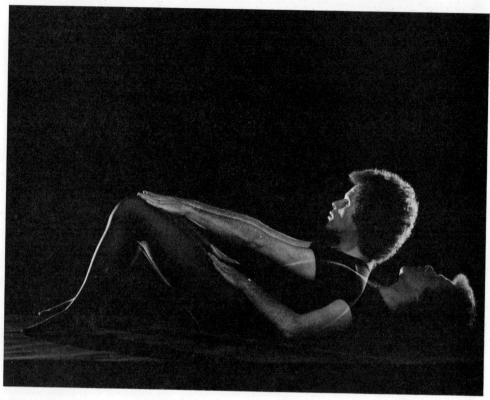

Mini Sit-ups
20

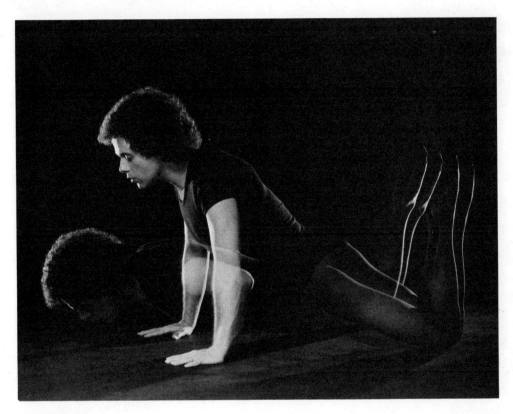

Mini Pushups
10

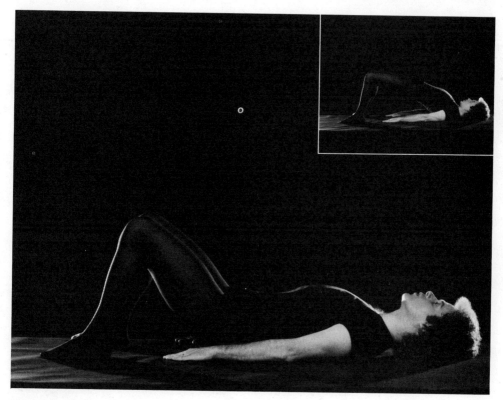

Buttocks Tucks
10

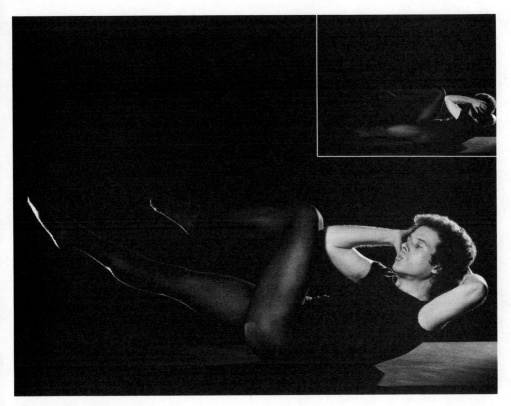

Knee to Elbow Bicycle Ride
30

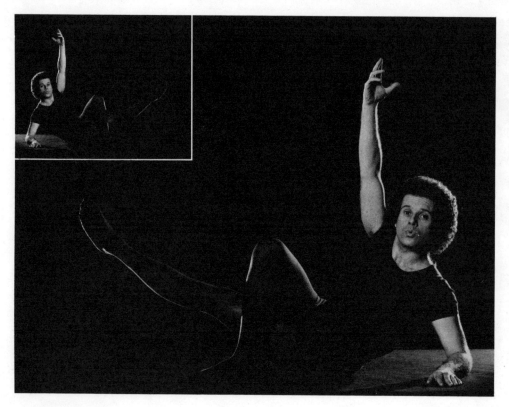

Inner Thigh Stretch
10 lifts with each leg

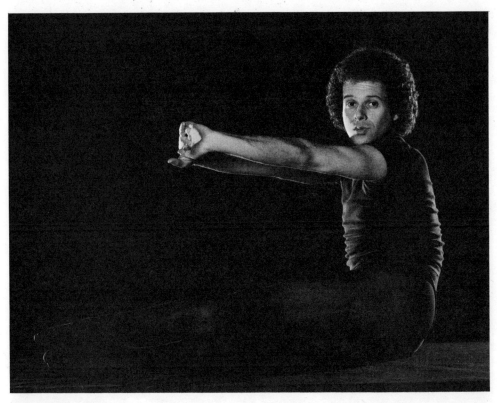

Tootsie Rolls
60/30 from cheek to cheek

If you are *twenty to forty pounds overweight* . . . you have nothing to worry about. You'll soon be out of the big numbers and into the teens. (And who doesn't want to be in the teens again?) The only way to whittle away the rest of your weight is to hang in there and bust your buns. You'll be home free soon!

The First Five Minutes Every Morning

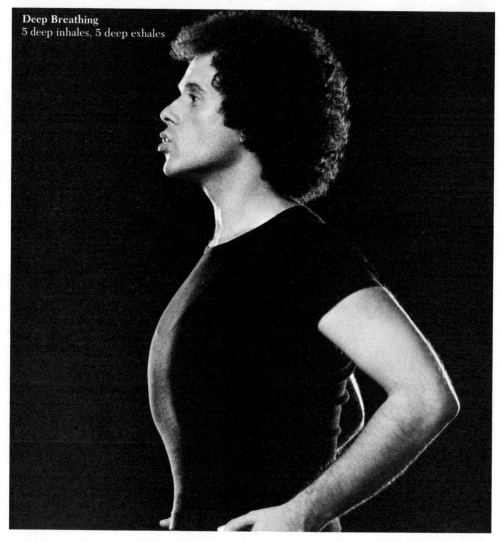

Deep Breathing
5 deep inhales, 5 deep exhales

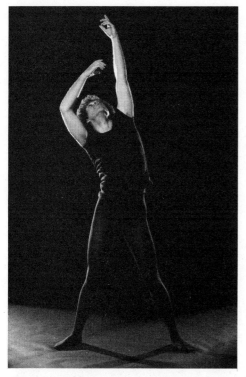 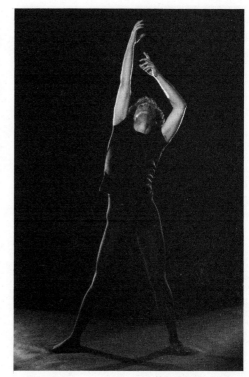

Climb and Stretch
30 climbs, 15 with each hand

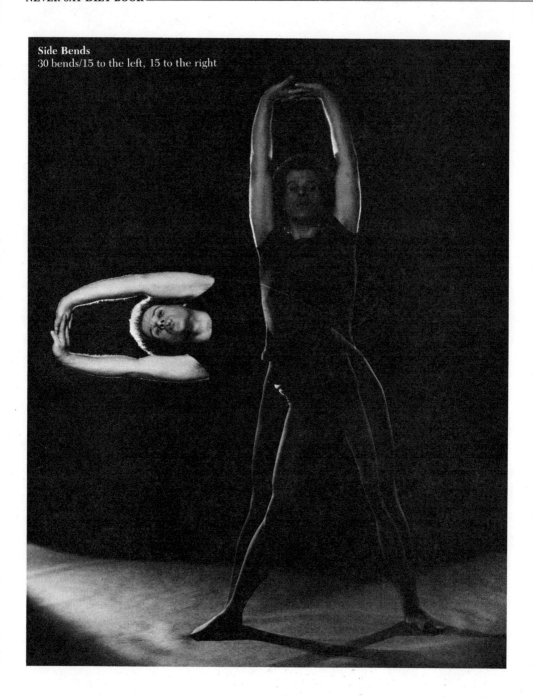

Side Bends
30 bends/15 to the left, 15 to the right

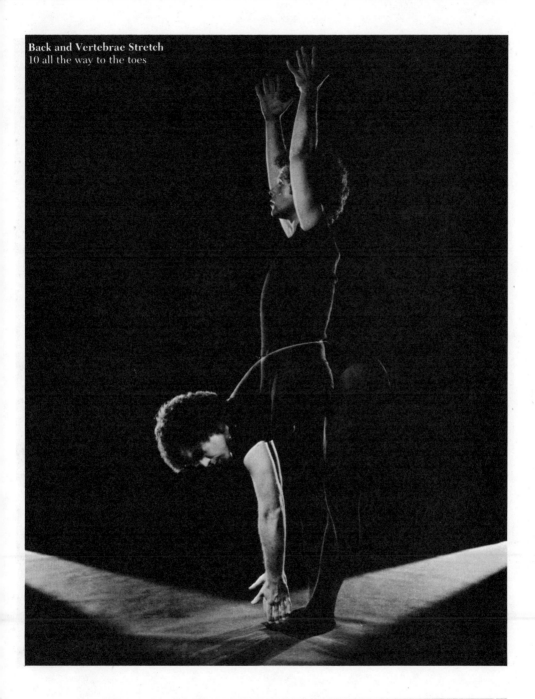

Back and Vertebrae Stretch
10 all the way to the toes

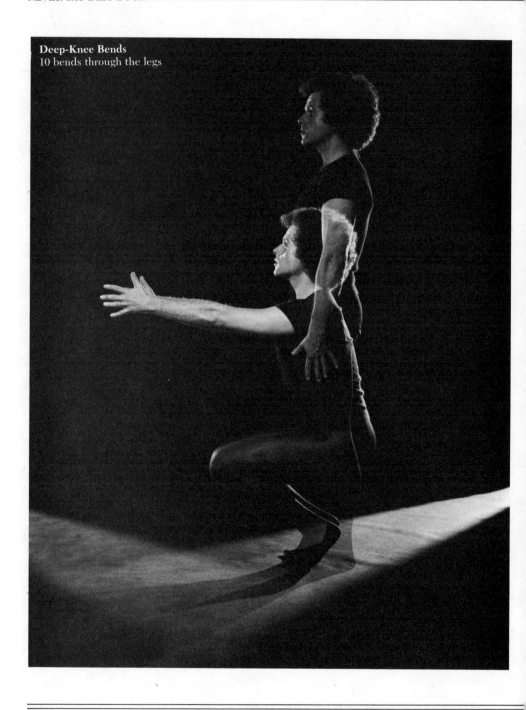

Deep-Knee Bends
10 bends through the legs

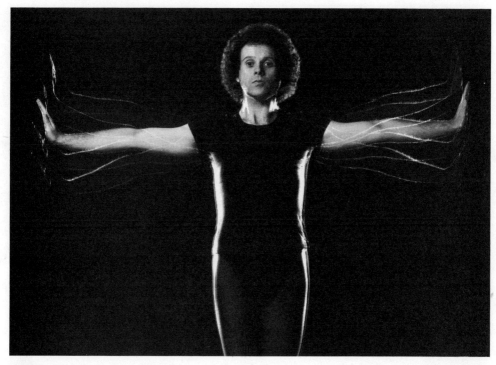

Arm Circles
15 clockwise, 15 counterclockwise

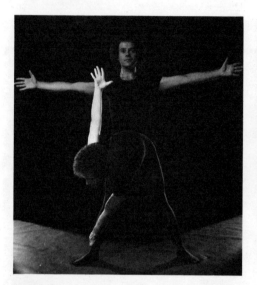 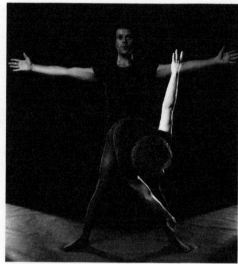

Toe to Toe
30 turns/15 to each foot

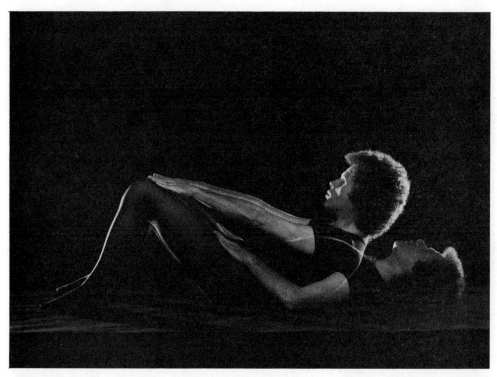

Mini Sit-ups
20

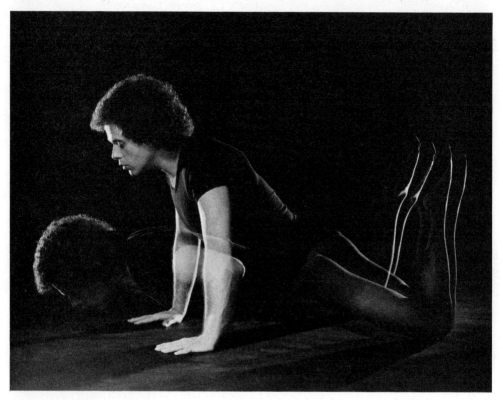

Mini Pushups
15

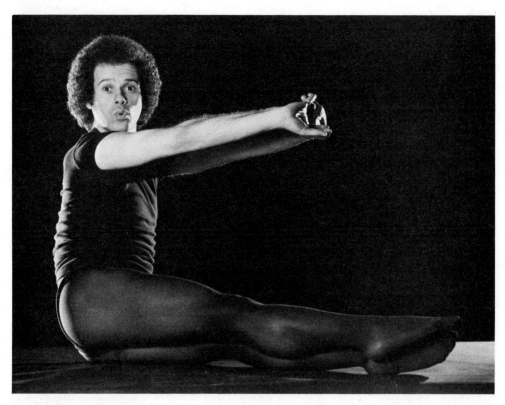

Tootsie Rolls
100, 50 from cheek to cheek

The Last Five Minutes in the Evening

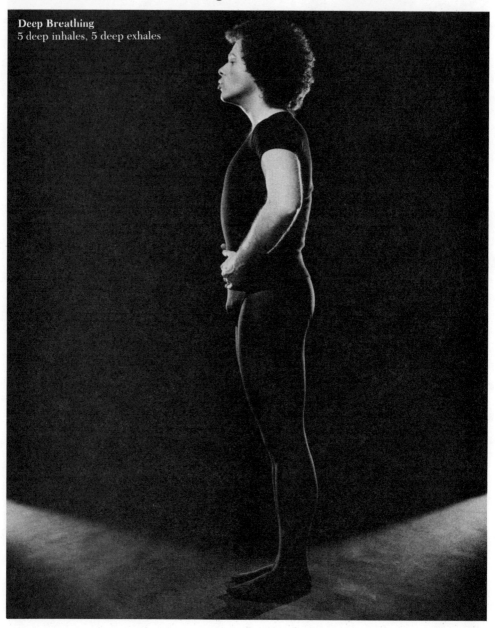

Deep Breathing
5 deep inhales, 5 deep exhales

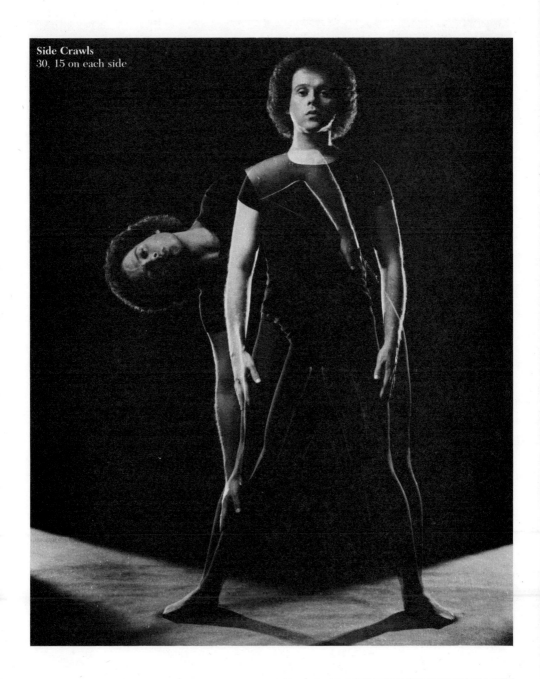

Side Crawls
30, 15 on each side

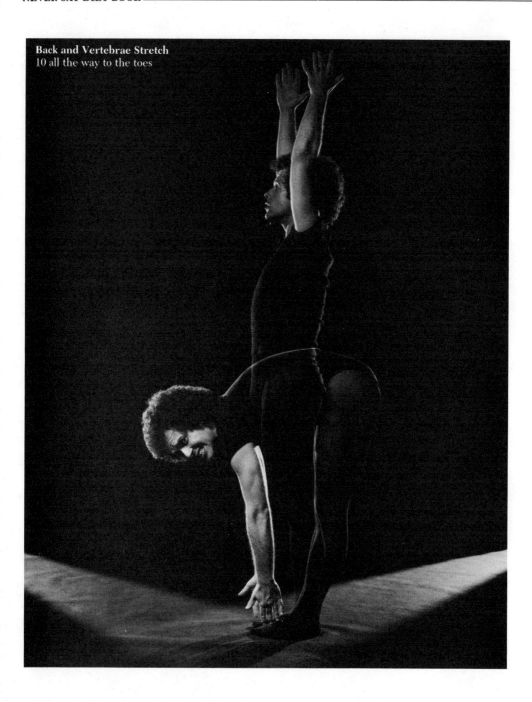

Back and Vertebrae Stretch
10 all the way to the toes

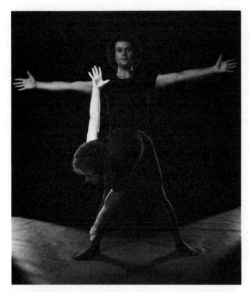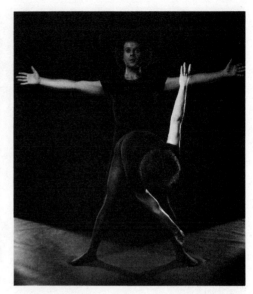

Toe to Toe
30 turns/15 to each foot

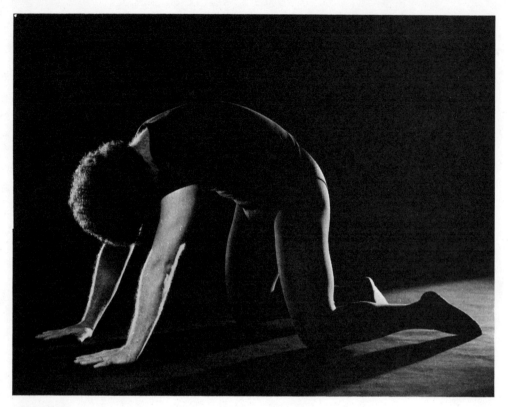

Cat Stretch
10 inhales, 10 exhales

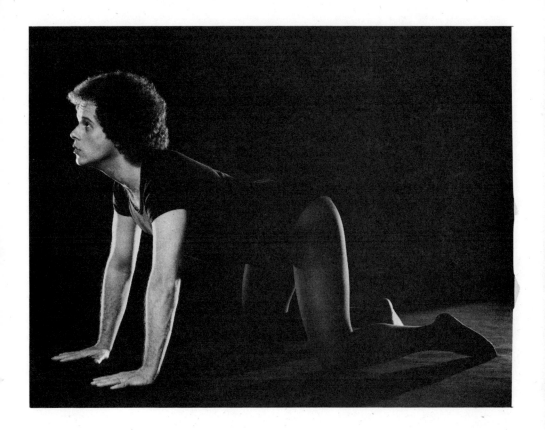

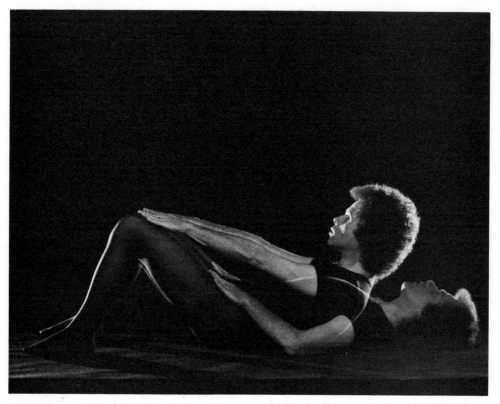

Mini Sit-ups
20

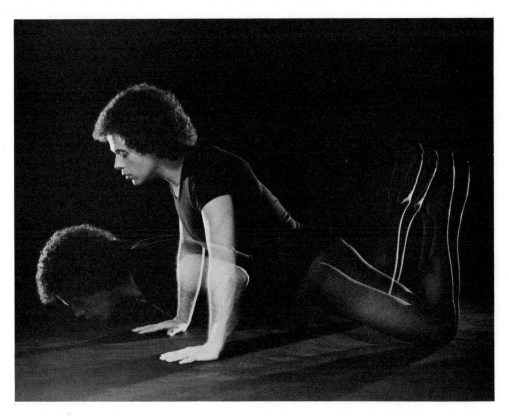

Mini Pushups
20

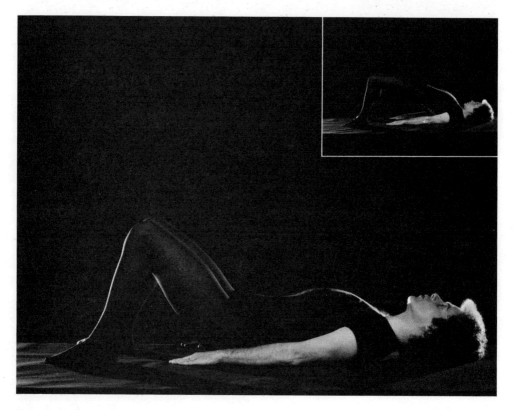

Buttocks Tucks
15

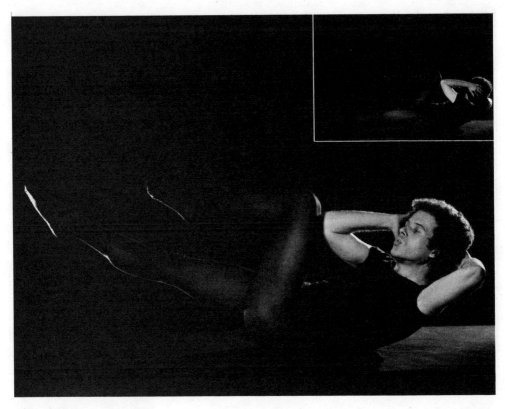

Knee to Elbow Bicycle Ride
30

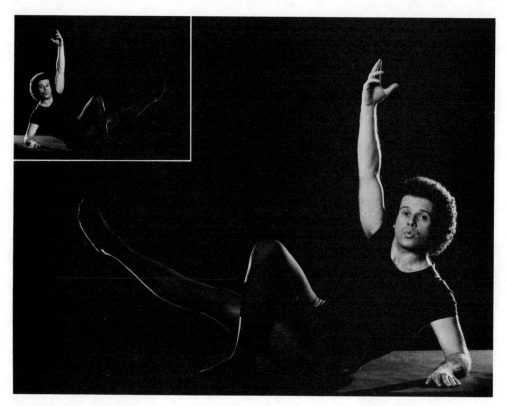

Inner Thigh Stretch
15 lifts with each leg

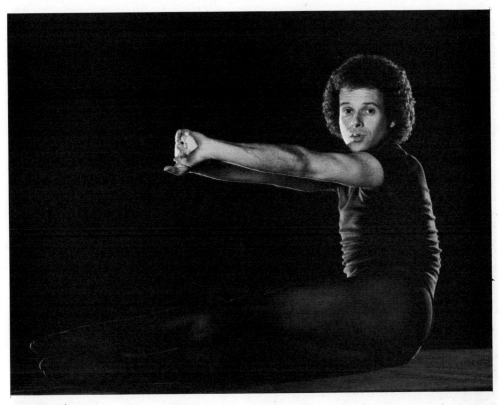

Tootsie Rolls
100/50 from cheek to cheek

If you are *zero to fifteen pounds overweight,* this combined set of exercises is going to show you just how easy it is to shape up all over your body. That flat stomach you wanted—it's yours. The inside of your leg—cottage-cheese lumps—gone forever. Discipline—don't forget that word—ever.

The First Five Minutes Every Morning

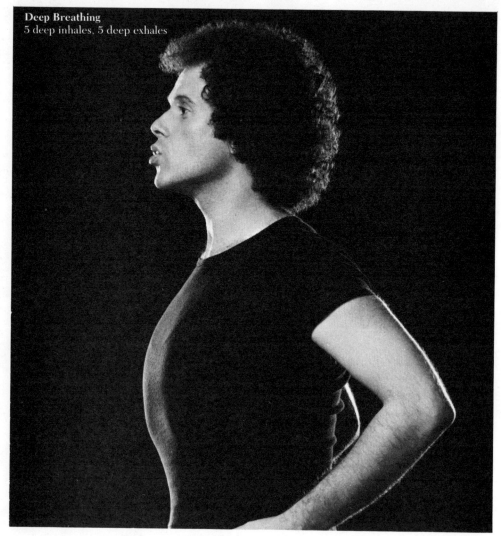

Deep Breathing
5 deep inhales, 5 deep exhales

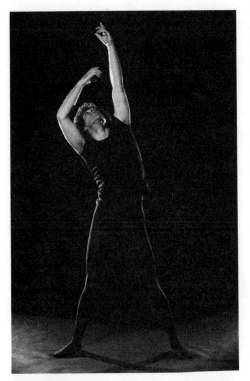 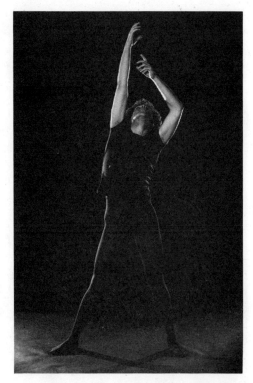

Climb and Stretch
50 climbs/25 with each hand

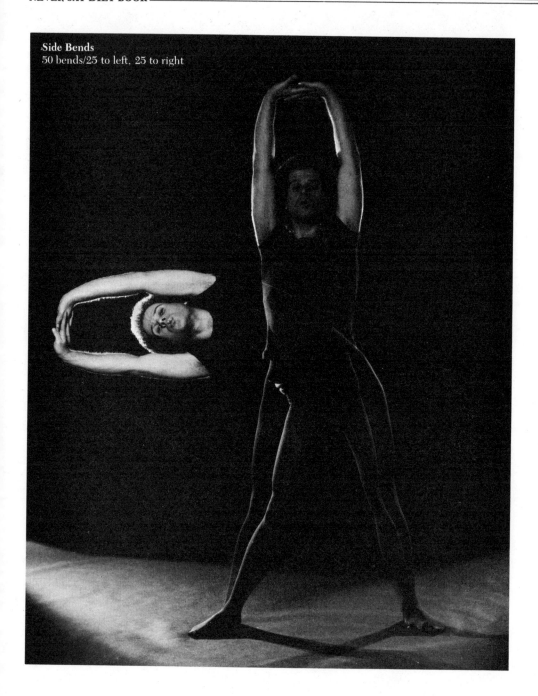

Side Bends
50 bends/25 to left, 25 to right

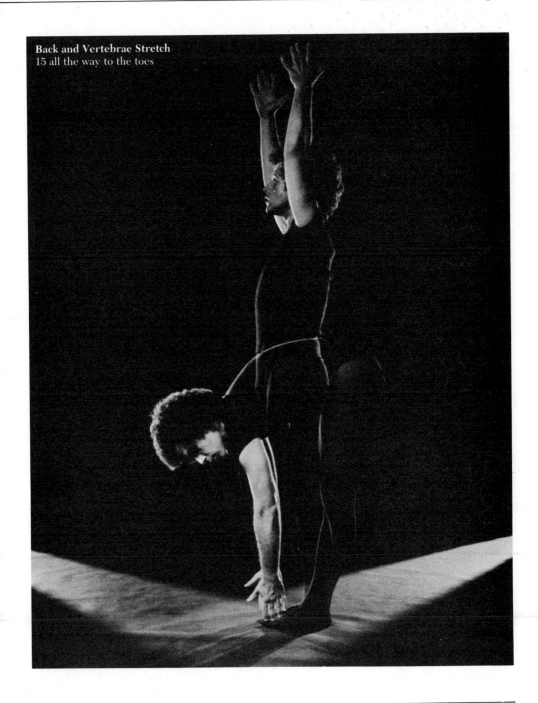

Back and Vertebrae Stretch
15 all the way to the toes

Deep-Knee Bends
15 bends through the legs

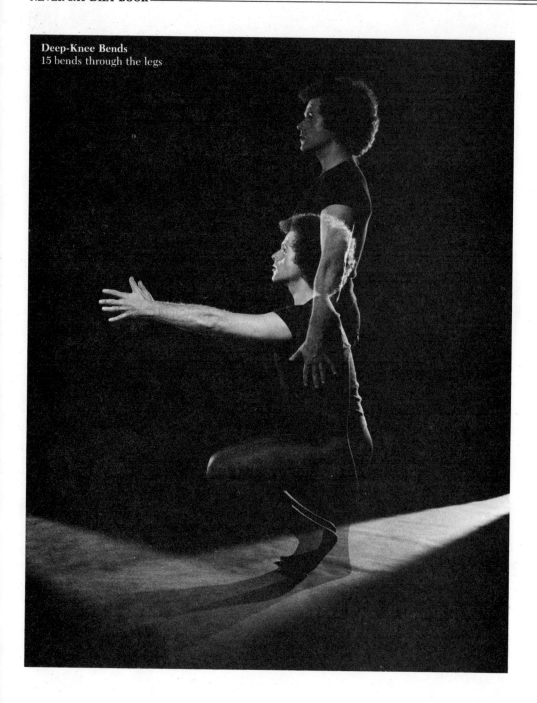

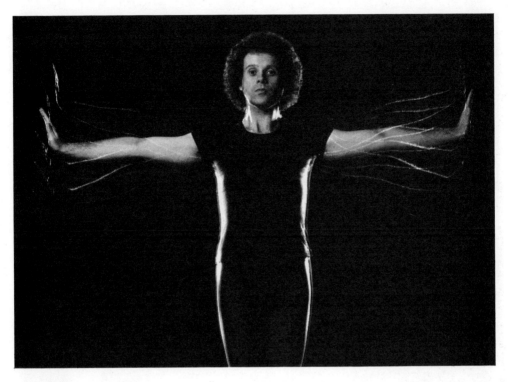

Arm Circles
25 clockwise, 25 counterclockwise

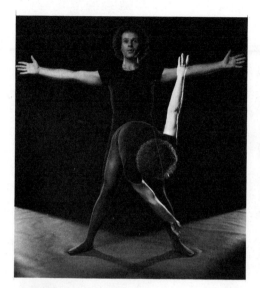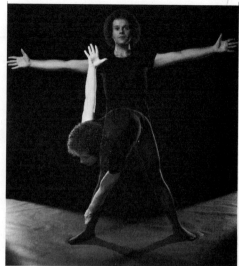

Toe to Toe
50 turns/25 to each foot

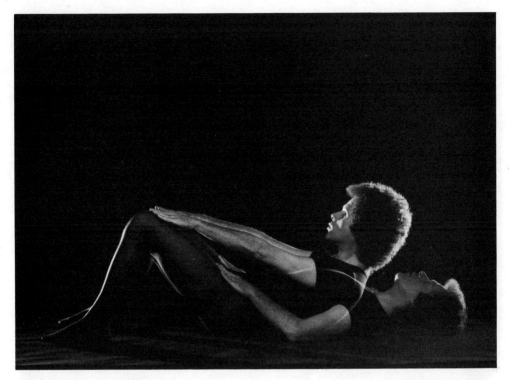

Mini Sit-ups
30

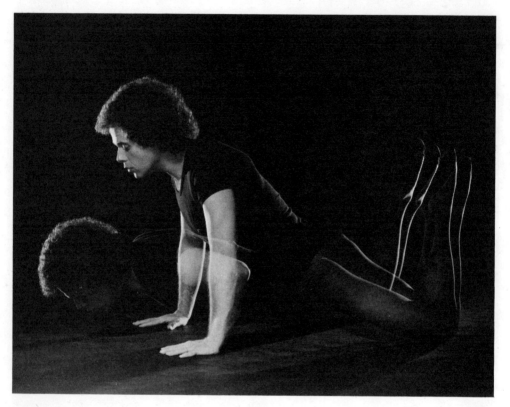

Mini Pushups
20

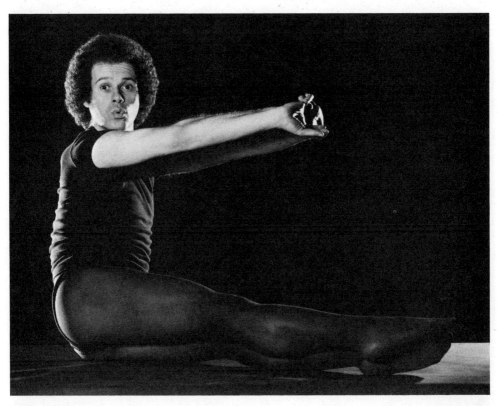

Tootsie Rolls
150, 75 from cheek to cheek

The Last Five Minutes in the Evening

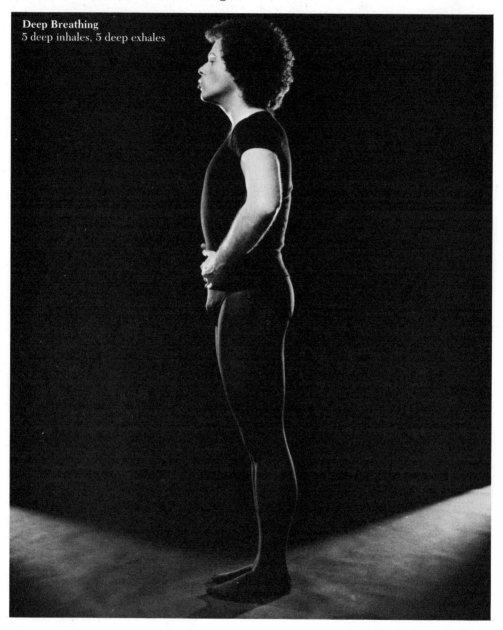

Deep Breathing
5 deep inhales, 5 deep exhales

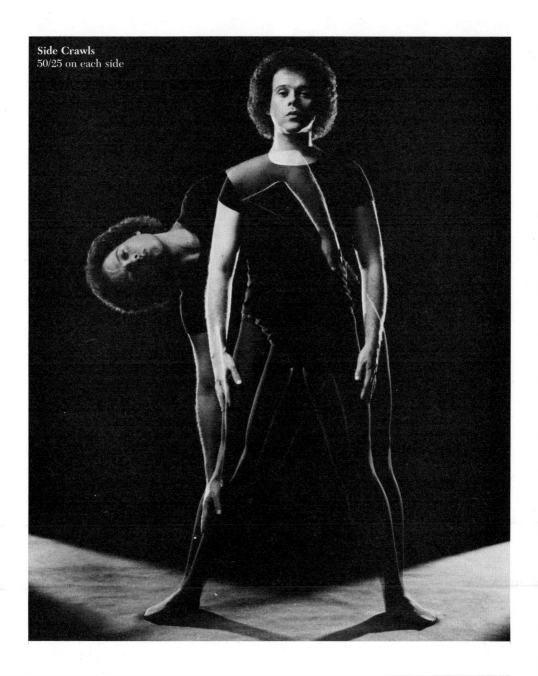

Side Crawls
50/25 on each side

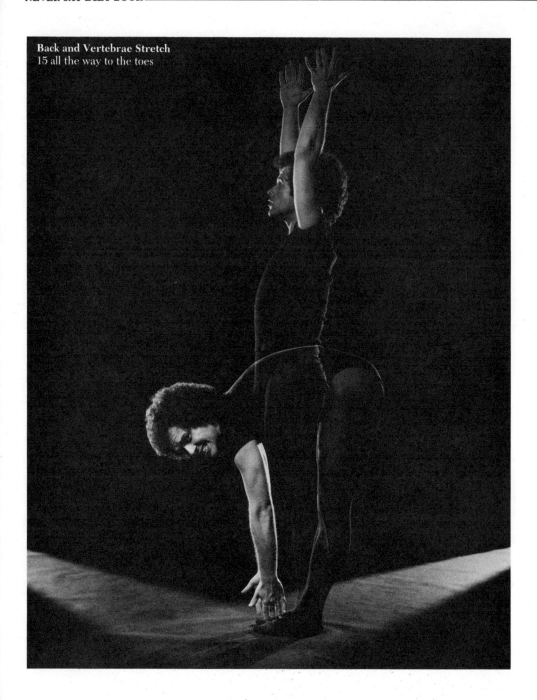

Back and Vertebrae Stretch
15 all the way to the toes

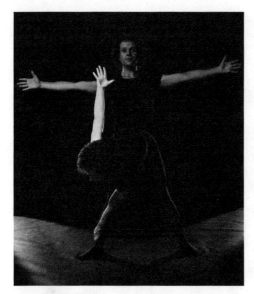 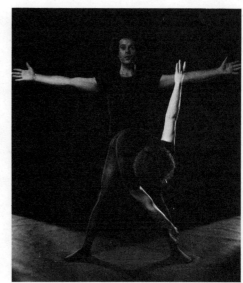

Toe to Toe
50 turns/25 to each foot

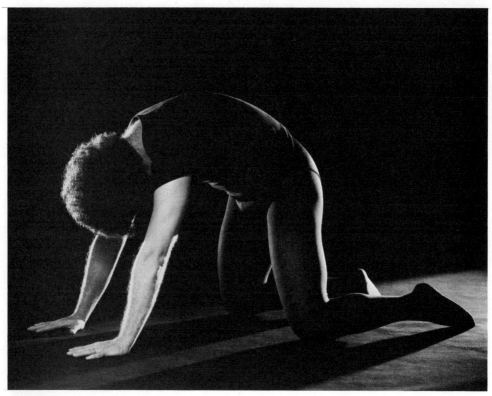

Cat Stretch
15 inhales, 15 exhales

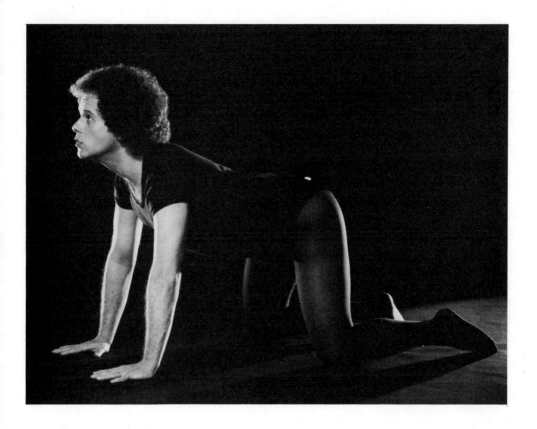

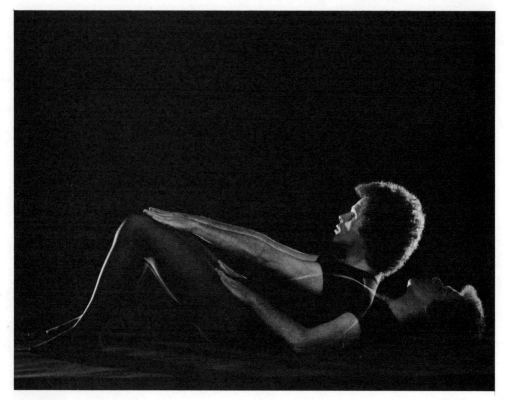

Mini Sit-ups
30

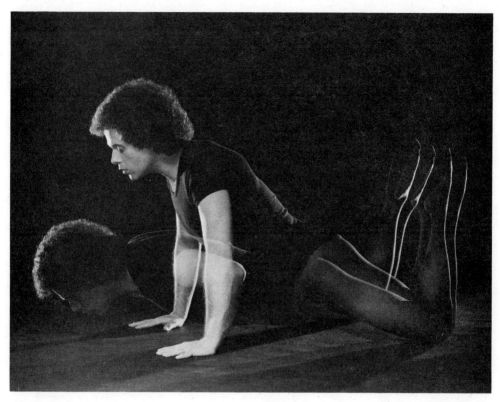

Mini Pushups
20

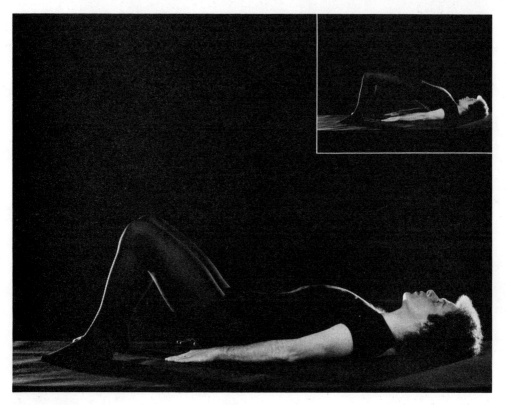

Buttocks Tucks
25

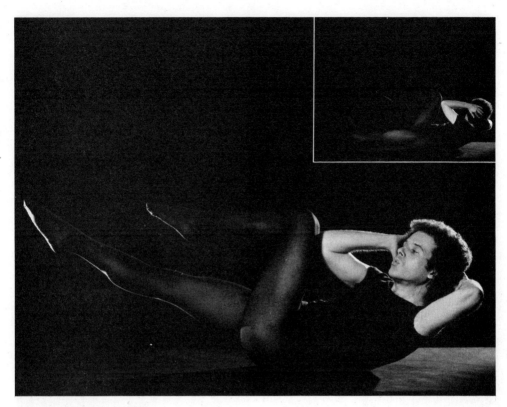

Knee to Elbow Bicycle Ride
50

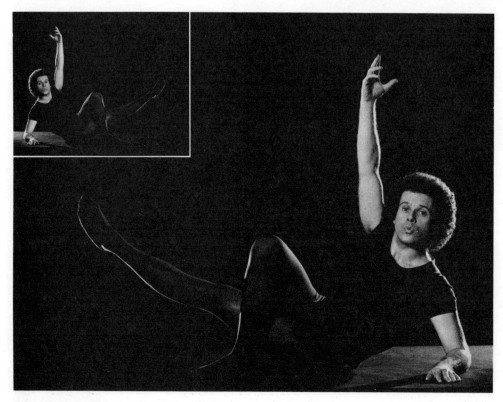

Inner Thigh Stretch
25 lifts with each leg

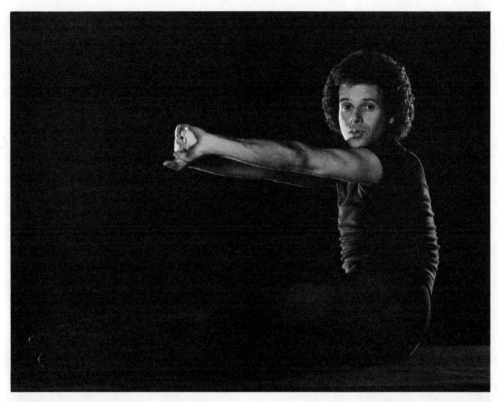

Tootsie Rolls
150/75 from cheek to cheek

By now you must be saying to yourself, "This guy must be a little wacky—I can't do these exercises in five minutes." Oh yes you can! At first you'll be looking at the pictures and reading how to do them, but in less than a week your Live-It Exercise Program will be second nature.

Don't forget the music. Turn on that radio or stereo, get involved in that music. I don't care if you love Andy Williams, Dolly Parton, or Bach. It doesn't matter. The beat, the tempo, and the voice makes exercise a whole lot more enjoyable. As I describe the movements to you I'll also include some of the music selections I use in my classes.

check your posture before beginning any of these exercises).

● Inhale through the nose, then let all the air out slowly. You are expanding your lungs and getting your heart started—there's no better way of beginning your morning than with proper breathing habits.

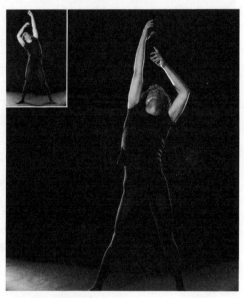

Climb and Stretch
● Stay in your standing position, feet apart. Hold your stomach in, lift your neck high, and look at the ceiling.

● Bring both hands above the head as if you're ready to climb a rope. Alternate your breathing as you shift your upper torso. Right-hand reach as you *inhale*, left-hand reach as you *exhale*.

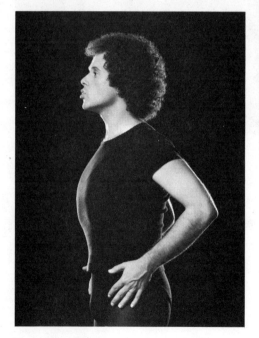

Deep Breathing
● Stand up straight, shoulders back, neck tall, and feet apart (remember always to

● You should feel all the pulling sensation in your shoulders and also from your waist (keep that stomach in, and tight).

• Just keep thinking about pulling that rope higher and higher. Come on, it's a rope, not a piece of dental floss.

◊ ◊ ◊

Side Bends

• Same position. This time lace your fingers together, elbows nice and straight, head up—stomach in.

• Inhale (through the nose) and S-L-O-W-L-Y exhale as you bend all the way to the left. Don't worry how low you can bend—it may take a while for your muscles to respond; besides, we know there's cheesecake or root-beer floats stored somewhere between your ribcage and your hip.

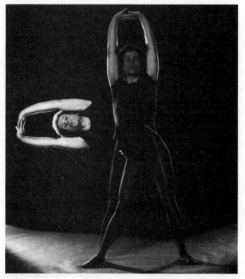

• Inhale as you S-L-O-W-L-Y take up the upper part of your body and repeat on the right side.

• These bends not only limber up your sides but also stretch your arms, chest, back, and neck areas.

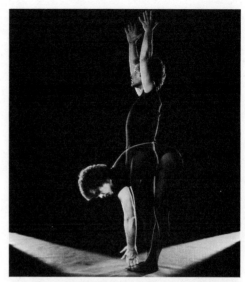

Back and Vertebrae Stretch

• Legs together please, stomach in, tighten your rear, and check your neck (always keep that chin up).

• Again, bring both hands above your head and spread your fingers wide—they need some air and exercise, too.

• Inhale and S-L-O-W-L-Y exhale as you begin your descent to your toes area. Now hold that stomach in. Inhale on the way back up and exhale as you go down again.

• This exercise stretches your whole back side—neck, shoulders, vertebrae , back, and legs. The muscles in your legs may be tight and getting all the way to the toes may seem impossible. Don't worry—they'll loosen up and stay firm.

◊ ◊ ◊

Deep-Knee Bends

• Now it's time to stretch your knees and the front and inside of your legs.

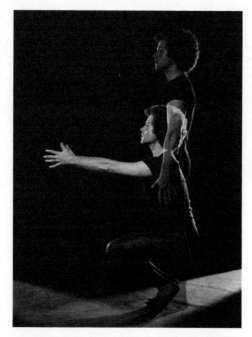

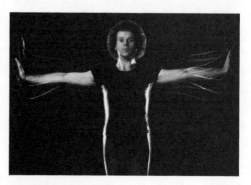

• Feet apart, give me your best posture. Come on, just think what that body of yours is gonna look like soon. Get those arms up above your head.

• Inhale and as you exhale bend your knees and take a dive between your legs pushing both hands through the leg opening. (Like Esther Williams in *Summer in the Everglades*.)

• Inhale and come up again, exhale and swing down there, keeping that stomach in tight. (Remember also to round your neck and head and to do these nice for Esther!)

◊ ◊ ◊

Arm Circles
• Legs tight, real tight, please. Chin up and smile. We're gonna make those arms slim and tight so that when you wave to

someone your whole arm doesn't jiggle around like a dish of Jell-O.

• Extend both arms, tighten them, and flatten the palms of your hands.

• Begin rotating your arms, at first with small circles, then working up to bigger ones. Keep a constant flow of air circulating through the lungs. Inhale through nose, exhale through mouth. Don't do this exercise to real fast music or you'll find yourself flying out the window.

• Remember, clockwise and counterclockwise.

◊ ◊ ◊

Toe to Toe
• Turn on one of those Herb Alpert and the Tijuana Brass albums and get in a Latin mood (not pig-Latin).

• Spread your feet wide. S-L-O-W-L-Y bend down as if you're removing gum from the front of your shoe.

• With your left hand touch your right foot and inhale. Switch, and now exhale as your right hand touches your left foot.

• Stay down low and keep switching from left to right, cha, cha, cha.

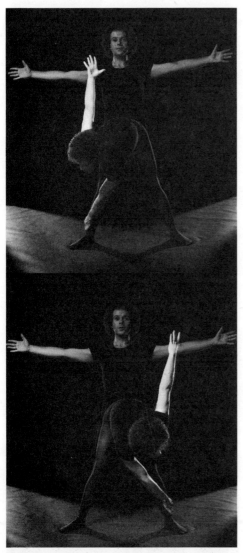

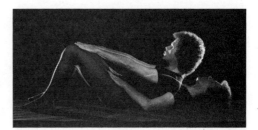

waistline, hips, and thighs, and also helps firm up the arms.

◇ ◇ ◇

Mini Sit-ups
● Lie down on the floor. (No, this is not a rest period—this is tummy period.) Bend your knees and spread your feet a bit.

● Rest your hands at the base of your legs. Inhale with your back and head flat on the floor. Exhale while you slowly glide up your legs all the way to your knee caps. Keep your chin tucked into your chest. Inhale as you go down.

● Believe me, this one is a killer at first. The thing this exercise does right away is make you aware of the fat around your stomach. You put it there and only you can get rid of it. And you will, I promise you. Now that news is something to sit up about! Remember, the slower you do these the more your fat cells will hate you.

◇ ◇ ◇

Mini Pushups
● Get on all fours like Lassie. Spread your knees and your hands about two feet apart.

● Make sure your head, neck, back, and tushy are on the same angle. This position releases any pressure from your back. Your arms and your chest will be doing all the work.

● Remember to keep the other arm high in the air, so while one arm is stretching down the other is stretching up—that's real balance.

● This is the greatest exercise for your

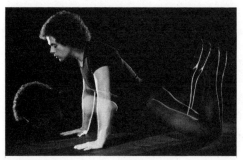

• Inhale in the up position (straight elbows—check your posture) and exhale as you slowly lower your body. Inhale and come up all the way back till your elbows are straight again.

• These are also tough at first, but don't give up. No, these pushups *will not* make your arms look like Hercules. That's nonsense. Nadia Comaneci, the famous gymnast, does five hundred of these every morning, and there's nothing bulky about her.

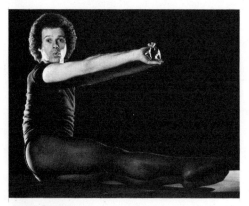

Tootsie Rolls
• Sit up straight, legs together tight, and extend your arms out again. Now all you have to do is lift up your rear one bun at a time and rock from side to side. ("Shall We

Dance," from the musical *The King and I*, is perfect music.)

• Inhale while lifting the right bun, exhale while lifting the left bun. Remember to lock those legs and lift those buns as high as you can.

• As your thighs, hips, and rear are bouncing from side to side, make sure that stomach is held in. And where's your neck? Good, nice and high.

Now, that wasn't so bad, was it? These simple stretches have activated your whole body. Every cell is just raring to go and have an up and positive day. When you begin your mornings with this ritual you're in total control.

And now for your evening stretches.

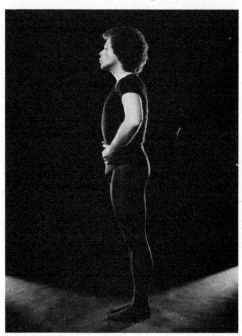

Deep Breathing

● I know you've had a hard day. These deep breaths will ease the tension. Close your eyes, if you like, and relax.

● Stand up straight, shoulders back, neck tall, feet apart.

● Inhale through the nose, then S-L-O-W-LY let all the air out of your lungs. In the evening do these much slower than the morning ones. Remember, you're unwinding.

◇ ◇ ◇

Side Crawls

● Straighten up, feet apart, hands to your side, neck up.

● Inhale and slowly exhale as you slide down the right side of your body. Come on, a little lower—you can do these. Inhale on the way up and exhale as you slide down the left side of your body. Just imagine yourself as a big oil rig drilling for oil. . . . Up. . . . Down. . . . Up. . . . Down. Inhale—Exhale. . . . Inhale—Exhale.

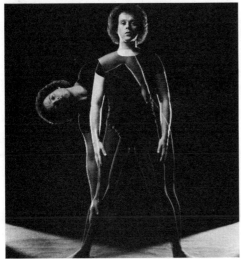

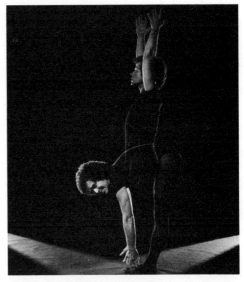

Back and Vertebrae Stretch

● Legs together, stomach in, tighten that rear. Bring both hands above your head. Remember to spread those fingers wide.

● Inhale and S-L-O-W-L-Y exhale as you stretch all the way down to your toes. Inhale as you come up, and try to feel every bone and every muscle working. During the day, while sitting at your desk or driving or just walking, you have a tendency to knock parts of your body out of whack. This exercise helps to loosen your neck and back area. Those tension knots will disappear, too.

◇ ◇ ◇

Toe to Toe

● I know how much you enjoyed these this morning, so here we go again. Spread those feet wide, bend down slowly, and with your left hand touch your right foot and inhale. Switch, and now exhale as your right hand touches your left foot.

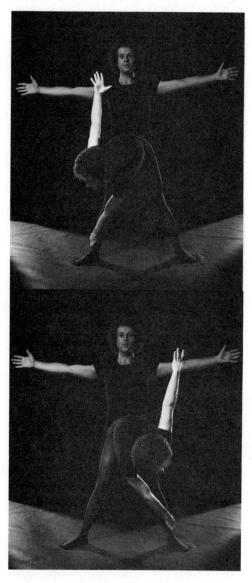

• Keep that rhythm going right, left—inhale, exhale. You won't get dizzy if you turn your head the same way and keep that other arm high in the air.

Cat Stretch

• Get on all fours. If your knees have a tendency to ache, slip a towel under them for cushioning purposes. Spread your legs just a bit and keep those elbows straight during the entire exercise.

• Flatten your back, sticking your rear up in the air, as well as your head, and inhale. Slowly let the air out as you drop your head into your chest area and arch your back as high as you can. Please hold your stomach in. If this exercise looks familiar to you it's because you've seen a cat stretch his back like this before.

• This one is simple if you remember to inhale when the neck and head are down, back is arched.

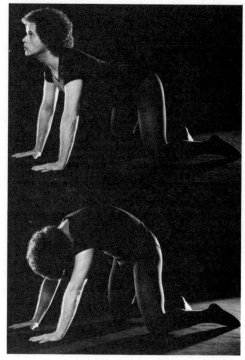

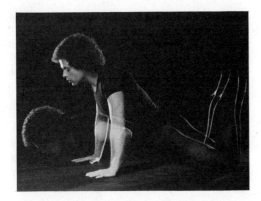

Mini Pushups

● Down on the knees and hands again, please. Spread your knees and hands about two feet.

● Don't forget to check your posture and also the angle of your body.

● Inhale in the up position and exhale as you slowly lower your body. Inhale again on the way up. You should look to the left and the right as you're doing these to see how your arms are working against gravity to burn off the fat and tone the muscles.

◇ ◇ ◇

Mini Sit-ups

● Lie down on the floor, spread your feet a bit, and bend the knees.

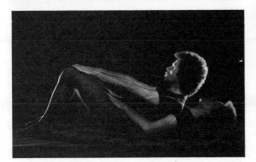

● Again rest your hand at the base of your legs. Inhale in this flat position and slowly climb up those legs till you reach the knee-caps. Inhale as you slowly release the tension in your stomach, and rest.

● Please concentrate on your breathing and think to yourself, "I'm toning and flattening my stomach so I'll have a nice profile."

◇ ◇ ◇

Buttocks Tucks

● Stay where you are with your knees bent, feet spread a bit, head and back flat on the floor. Put your hands at your sides.

● Inhale as you lift your rear up off the ground, tightening the buttocks in the up

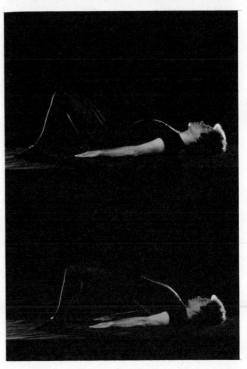

position. Hold for a count of five tight—as tight as you can.

● Exhale S-L-O-W-L-Y on your way down.

● This is a very sexy exercise so might as well have music to match—Carly Simon singing "Nobody Does It Better."

● Make sure everything is relaxed—your neck, hands, and arms—and let your behind do all the work. You see, the rear doesn't do much beside sit, stand, and lie. This exercise pushes it up against gravity while tightening and firming the thighs, hips, and bottom.

IMPORTANT!
Hold your stomach in as tight as you can. Concentrate and do these very S-L-O-W-L-Y.

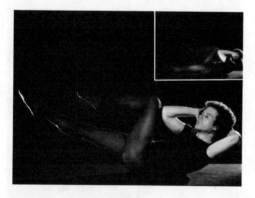

Knee to Elbow Bicycle Ride
● This one is an old army exercise. You can do it to "Stout-Hearted Men" or "Over There." It's for the waist, stomach, hips, thigh, leg, arm, back, and neck areas. This exercise does nothing for the elbow . . . I'm sorry.

● Lie on your back, lace your hands behind your head, twist your body so your left

elbow touches your right knee, and inhale while doing this.

● Then twist your torso the other way so your right elbow touches your left knee as you exhale.

● Please constantly check your posture. Are your hands supporting your head, neck, and upper back? Are your toes pointed? Are you lowering the legs as low as you possibly can? Are you breathing and turning your head as your body twists?

◇ ◇ ◇

Inner Thigh Stretch
● Lie on your side, balancing on one elbow and keeping the other arm high in the sky. Cross your right leg over your left and bend it at the knee. Inhale and slowly lift your

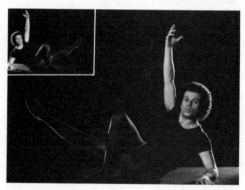

left leg (point those toes). Exhale as you slowly let the leg down.

● Make sure your back is straight and your chin is up. This is the best over-all exercise for that mushy thigh area.

● When you've completed the number of lifts you've been assigned, turn around, cross your left leg over your right, and bend at the knee. Start lifting your right leg the same way.

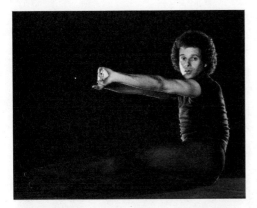

Tootsie Rolls

● I know you love these, so we'll do them one more time before we put your hips to bed.

● Sit up. Straight back, legs together tight, extend arm, and start lifting that rear, one bun at a time.

● Inhale, right bun—exhale, left bun. If you are in a room with good light pick up a magazine, keep your arms extended, and read while you rock—I hope you're not nearsighted. This takes your mind off the exercise and most probably you'll be able to do a thousand of these in no time. Please don't read cookbooks. Exercise and drooling are not a good combination.

When you have pretty much mastered your Live-It Exercise Program (that should take two weeks), you'll be able to try a few good-ies for problem areas and a few advanced versions of the exercises you've been doing. Take your time, though, and remember these points:

CONCENTRATE: You've gotten this far, so go all the way. Keep on saying to yourself, "Do you want a healthy body or not?" If you do, stop complaining and keep on trucking.

CHECK YOUR POSTURE: Support all your internal organs by holding in that stomach. Keep that back straight and your head up. By continually checking your body before you start exercising, maximum results will be achieved.

LET THE AIR TAKE YOU WHERE YOU WANT TO GO: You must be sick of hearing me mention breathing, but I must keep reminding you of its importance.

REST BUT NEVER SKIP AN EXERCISE: If you have to stop for a moment, then stop. Don't skip an exercise you don't like or think you don't need. Remember, it's the combination of these exercises that's going to get you in shape. Your body must work as a single unit.

Are Your Arms and Chest the Pits?

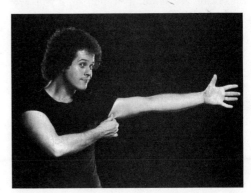

Put your right arm out and with your other hand feel the skin around your upper arm and chest area. Ugh! What you are feeling is fat and some tired muscle and skin. Remember what you don't use you lose. If you haven't been using all the parts of your arm you will lose tone and a certain degree of strength. *Isometric Exercises* are perfect for your arms and your chest, too. You will be using the strength in your arms and chest to pull against air and *gravity*.

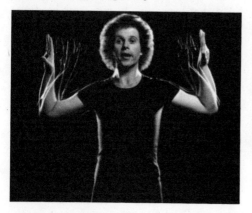

• Put your hands up (eye level) as if you're being arrested. Face the palms of your hand outward and pretend that two large walls of chocolate are coming at you and you are pushing them away.

• Inhale through the nose and slowly exhale as you push. Come on, push harder, or your head will get squished to death by the chocolate bars.

• After all the air has left your inside, return your hands closer to your ears. Inhale again, and this time push a lot harder as you exhale. Please keep your neck up and your stomach in.

• Repeat this exercise *ten* times.

◇ ◇ ◇

• Now keep your hands up and this time face the palms inward. It's as if some loud music is playing and you are trying to cover your ears, but something is holding you

back (that something is the strength in your arms and chest).

• Inhale and start pushing in, but resist . . . resist more as you exhale. Donna Summer is screaming in your ears, but you just

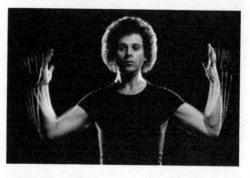

can't get to them.

• Repeat this exercise *ten* times.

◇ ◇ ◇

• Imagine you are lifting a very heavy box (no, not a fifty-pound box of candy).

• Inhale and push up with your hands as you exhale. You will feel a shaking sensation, but keep pushing upward until you're all out of air.

• Lift *ten* times.

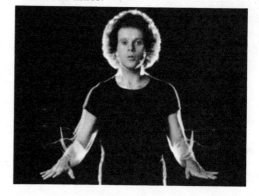

● Now you are pressing down on the box, so your palms are face down, of course.

● Inhale (is your stomach in)?

● S-L-O-W-L-Y exhale as you push downward.

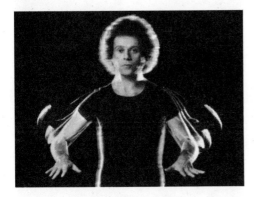

● Repeat this exercise *ten* times.

◊ ◊ ◊

During these isometrics remember at all times to keep a straight back and your chin up, relax the muscles in your face, and spread the fingers as wide as possible.

*Let's Face It*_____

Do you have to face it? No, not really. But if you have worked hard firming up the muscles in your body, don't you think the muscles in your face also need a workout?

Quick, get a mirror—and don't tell me you don't have one.

Look at your face and your neck. Well, what do you think? What's going through your mind as you stare at a big part of you? That you've neglected these areas?

◊ ◊ ◊

1. "It looks like a road map; where did all those lines come from?"

2. "I really don't know what happened. I look so puffy and distorted."
3. "I have to admit I look a lot better in pictures. Guess it's because all that light flashes in my face."

If you think gravity pulls down on your body, multiply that pulling force by ten and that's what's happening to that baby face and neck of yours.

Sagging skin and lines are indications that certain muscles are not being used. We've talked about constant movement in the body—well, the face needs constant correct movement also.

Will all the lines in your face and neck disappear? No. Can some of the loose skin firm up a bit and give your face more tone? Yes. Can you look years younger without surgery? Absolutely.

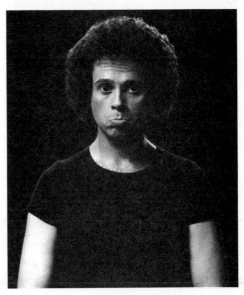

Pout-ers
● Now hold your head up high and pout.

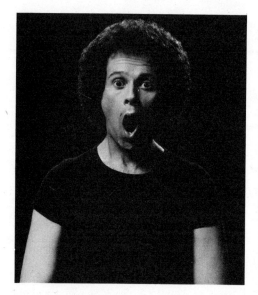

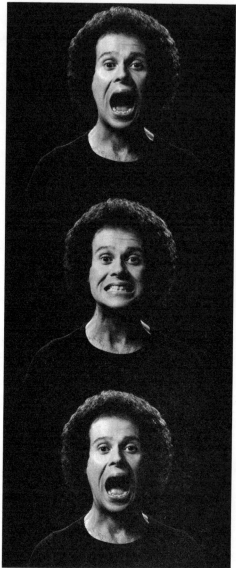

• Don't tell me you don't know how to pout—you didn't gain that weight by saying no. Like me, you usually pouted until you got what you wanted.

• You are now going to tone up your chin and mouth area. Inhale through the nose as you pout, then drop your chin all the way down and exhale through the mouth.

• Repeat the pout *ten* times.

Chew-Man-Chew

• Head up again. This time open your mouth and start chewing (straighten that back and hold that stomach in. No one's at ease yet).

• Come on, chew wider, exaggerate a bit. You also didn't get that shape by taking small bites.

• Keep that head up and chew. This is the only time you have ever chewed without gaining weight. Air is very dietetic, you know.

• *Twenty-five* nice, big chews, please.

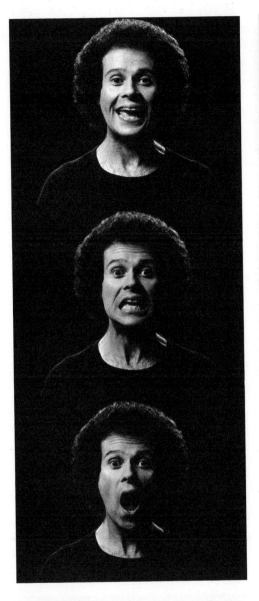

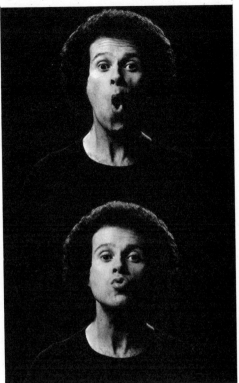

(and we know how important those areas are for eating).

● Look straight into the mirror, rest your eyebrows and forehead. Just concentrate on what's going on below the nose.

● Say the letter "A." It's a big smile, with your teeth a little forward.

● Hold your stomach in and get the sound of "A" out loud and clear.

● Inhale deep through the nose and exhale the vowel you are saying along with all the air.

● With "E" the corners of the mouth are

Vowel Stretchers

Remember, A-E-I-O-U? They work all the muscles around your neck and mouth pulling downward a bit, so most of your bottom teeth are showing.

● As you pronounce "I" elongate your face and drop your jaw.

● Pull all the way from your ears as you say "O." Start out with a big wide "O" and finish with a small one. Your jaw is still lowered doing the next vowel.

● "U" looks a little like a goldfish kissing the bowl. Your upper and lower lips protrude with your jaw and lower teeth pushed forward.

● So—you inhale through the nose and pronounce the vowels one by one while you exhale a little air out between them.

● Ready. Inhale and "A" (exhale) "E" (exhale) "I" (exhale) "O" (exhale) "U" (exhale). Good!

● Repeat *five* times and pay close attention to what's happening in the neck area. You are toning those muscles!

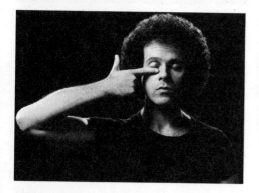

Under-Eye Tones
● This next one is so easy, you'll love it! It tightens the skin under your eye where bags and lines find a home.

● Close your eyes and relax all muscles on your face.

● While they are closed, without moving your eyebrows or forehead lift the eyeballs inside the closed lids upward.

● Take your index finger and place it gently under the eye areas so you can feel the muscles working.

● Now keep those eyes closed and lift the inside eyeball again. Do you feel that pull? Well, that pull is toning up those under-eye areas.

● And you thought I was just pulling your eye.

● Be careful, now. Don't poke your finger in your eye, please.

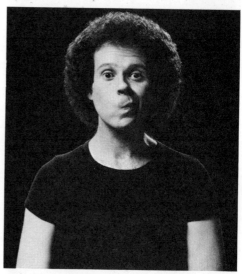

Wrinkle Wipes
● These aren't particularly attractive, but neither are chubby jowls and chubby chins. Those small lines that keep getting deeper

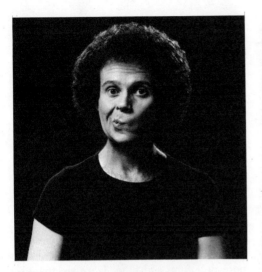

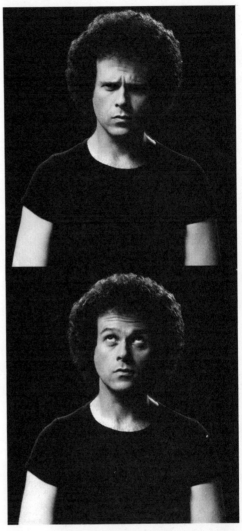

and deeper aren't so pretty, either.

● Your inhaling and exhaling will be done through the nose because the mouth is closed.

● Inhale and turn your lips all the way to the right side of your face. Hold it there and exhale. Inhale and come back to center, turn your lips all the way to the left side of your face, and exhale.

● *Five* wipes on each side.

◇ ◇ ◇

Frown and Stretch
● Pull your eyebrows down and close together. Hold for a count of three (one–two–three).

● Lift your eyebrows high and open your eyes as wide as you can.

● One of the reasons you get lines on your forehead is that you lift your brow and wrinkle your forehead more than the opposite pull, so the balance of your muscles is off.

● Set these straight and do *twenty-five* brow stretches.

◇ ◇ ◇

Facial massages, chin straps, and clay—cement masks may bring the blood to your face and give it a glow, but only you can tone your face. Gravity does pull downward, and there are many other elements that cause wrinkles, lines, and over-all aging to the face and neck.

The sun. Isn't a tan pretty? Your skin is so brown and beautiful and dry! And when the tan fades away, what do you have? Right! Little teeny, fine lines—but they could be the start of something big. Because tiny lines become wrinkles in time. Sun blocks and suntan lotion, oils and creams help a bit, but anyone who adores the sun will get lines quicker than the ones who just don't make a big habit of lying out in those harmful rays for hours.

Wind, snow, and other weather elements. Also dry the skin and break down its elasticity. Since the skin on your face is a bit thin, you should protect it when you are out in bad weather.

Not wearing your glasses. And constantly squinting your eyes wrinkles your brow. Pulling your mouth up and distorting your smile lines makes for permanent indentations. If you hate your glasses, get contacts. If you hate glasses and contacts, you are in deep trouble and deep wrinkles.

Smoking. The mechanics of inhaling smoke from a cigarette causes tiny lines around your mouth area. The habit of smoking itself discolors skin, breaks down tissue fiber in your face and body, and doesn't do much for the whites of your eyes, either.

Drinking. Breaks tiny veins in your skin called capillaries. So little red lines run all through your face. Attractive, isn't it? Drinking causes puffiness around your eye area, and all that drinking is just no good for the pores.

Lack of sleep. Shows in your face more than anywhere else. There's no glow to the skin, no life, just a lot of bags and an over-all droopy look.

Worry. Also shows first in your face. But after exercising your body and your face, what's to worry about?

Advanced Exercises for the Danger Zones

Stomach, hips, thighs, legs, and rear. There you have them. The fatty five. The real troublemakers. Through the Live-It Exercise Program you will begin to see some incredible changes in your shape. Your waist won't be melting into your hips. You'll see more definition and tone. Here are five exercises that are a bit harder, and in about six weeks you may add them to your individual exercise program.

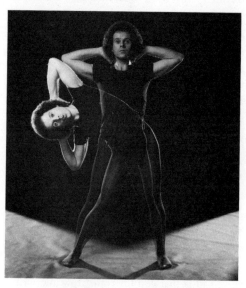

A Star Is Bending
● Place hands in back of your head (Mr.

DeMille, I'm ready for my close-up).

● Hold stomach in, inhale, and while exhaling slowly bend your torso down to the right as far as possible (let all the air out and go down as far as you can without falling over).

● Inhale on the way up and start heading down your left side while exhaling. You will be able to bend down lower on one side than the other: the P.E. teacher in high school said it depended on whether you were left-handed or right-handed. Whatever the reason be, it's true, so don't think you're lopsided—it's natural. *20 bends* on each side and Mr. DeMille says you can take a break!

Stomach Stretchers
● Lie down and prop yourself up on your

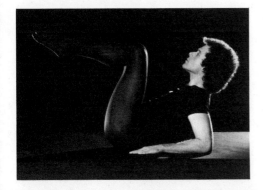

elbows. Bend your legs at the knee, point those toes, keep that chin up, and get ready, stomach.

● Inhale with the legs bent and slowly, very slowly, straighten your legs, keeping them as low to the floor as possible—the lower the better.

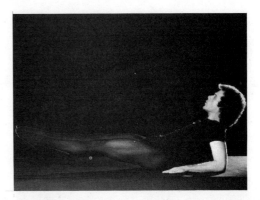

● Please, use the muscles in your stomach without help from the back, shoulders, and neck.

● You may want to put a towel up against your rear for this one. There's this little bone at the end of your spine that sticks out a bit and may have a tendency to hurt after a while. What? You don't have that bone? *20* stomach stretchers for now. You should be able to work up to 50.

Just Pulling Your Leg
● Roll over on your side and lift your right leg up; grab that ankle and lift as far as you can go. Your flexibility will get better, don't worry.

● Check your posture. Chin up, stomach in, straight back.

● Inhale (through the nose, remember) and slowly lift your left leg (the one on the floor) up so it can say hello to your other leg already up there. Exhale as you slowly let your left leg back down.

● This stretch affects your entire leg, from the pointed toes on up. At first you may not be able to lift that leg up too high. So

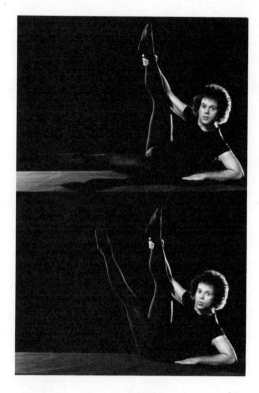

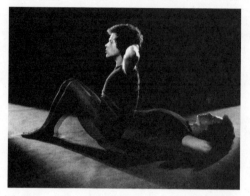

what—you got to start somewhere. Come on, practice makes a perfect set of legs.

• Turn the other way, grab the left leg, and slowly lift the right one. *20* lifts with each leg, and give your ankles a great big kiss.

◇ ◇ ◇

Advanced Sit-up
• Now stop using the word "hate"—it doesn't become you. I know these aren't your favorites, but I know you need them.

• Lie down on the floor, keep your legs together, and bend them at the knees. If I were you I'd put that towel back by the rear again.

• Lace your fingers in back of your head. Inhale in the flat position and exhale hard as your upper torso lifts up to a straight back. Inhale on the way back down.

• Strong breathing is essential for these sit-ups. Begin with ten, and thirty would be awful nice, don't you think?

Nose to Knee
• Here's a great stretch for your middle and those sides of yours.

• Sit up nice and straight. Extend your arms out and spread your legs as far as you can. Don't bend those knees—keep them straight.

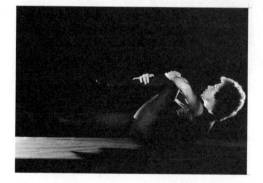

● Inhale in the up position. Take your left hand and wrap it around your right ankle while exhaling. Inhale on your journey back to your first position. Now take your right hand and wrap it around your left ankle while exhaling. These criss-cross numbers may sound difficult, but it's very similar to the exercise in your Live-It Program called Toe to Toe.

● Start off very slow. *20* noses to each knee, thank you kindly.

Well, we've exercised your lips, hips, elbows, and nose. We worked on your breathing, your posture, and that rear of yours. Have we left anything out? You bet your belly button! You need to learn how to exercise good eating habits and be mentally aware of what your body needs, inside and out.

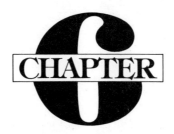

THE LIVE-IT FOOD PROGRAM

INTRODUCTION

I named this the *Never-Say-Diet Book* because if you follow my plan, you'll never use that dirty word again. And that's not a boast one can make idly. In fact, this isn't a diet book at all—but if I had called it *The Live-It Book* you probably wouldn't have bought it. And if you plunked down your hard-earned money for this book, chances are you need my help.

So here goes.

Remember that my plan is a three-way proposition. We're now at part two: The Live-It Food Plan that will accompany your daily exercise plan for the rest of your life. This isn't one of those silly diets that allows you two raisins as a treat and insists you

subsist on mangoes forever, so calm down. It is a healthy plan with a variety of foods that will allow you to maintain a regular lifestyle for the rest of your life. I think those contrived two-week diets are crazy. Where are you at the end of the two weeks? Or two weeks after that?

I have tested the Live-It Program (all three parts) over the past three years. I did not test it on white rabbits, brown mice, or baby chimps. I went for the real thing—overweight people. And if it worked for them, it will work for you. (Unless you are a white rabbit. . . .) Doctors, nutritionists, even psychiatrists sent me clients who had nothing physically wrong with them except for the fact that they couldn't drop the weight they needed to lose.

Why send these people to me? Because I was fat; I suffered through all the crap an overweight person has to deal with on an everyday level, but I beat it and I won. That's right, I won. I lost the weight. I kept it off and I've never had to read another diet book again. Now it's your turn.

Just one other thing to remember before you now take on part two of my program—if you have more than fifty pounds to lose, please consult your doctor first.

THE LIVE-IT FOOD PROGRAM

The Live-It Food Program offers a safe, balanced choice of foods to fill your day. No, there aren't a whole bunch of rules you have to follow: this is not a game. You're not going to win a washer/dryer or a trip to Hawaii. The variety of foods is generous (thank you very much) and you get to do the picking just as if you were reading a menu in a Chinese restaurant—you know, one from Column A, one from Column B, and so on. You don't have to eat Brussels sprouts on Mondays and cabbage on Fridays. You don't have to count calories, carbohydrates—you count nothing. Nor do you measure. What you do have to watch and be concerned with is the volume—the amount you are about to consume. When I say "a portion of chicken" you may have to reevaluate what "portion" means to you. (If you are overweight, then it's obvious you've been eating too big a portion, too often.) No one needs to finish off three breasts and five drumsticks in one sitting! One breast, without skin, is a portion—a thigh and a drumstick is fine, but ten chicken wings is too much. When you put carrots on your plate, tilting the serving dish over and emptying it out isn't necessary, a few tablespoons is plenty.

A person who is fifty or sixty pounds overweight has been eating a certain amount of food over a period of time in order to have accumulated those excessive pounds. Now, someone who is only ten pounds over has been generally eating far less food. What this means simply is that you gain weight when you overeat. The more you overeat, the more weight you gain. That's a medical and physiological fact. With this in mind—plus a little common sense—I base my program on this theory:

People who are at different weight levels should have a food plan to follow that has been designed for how much weight they have to lose. The degree of the weight problem is different—the rate at which a person will lose the weight is different, so the menus should be different, and they are. The same philosophy applies to helping the outside of the body with exercise. These plans are also designed for people with different degrees of weight. Someone who is really overweight doesn't have the same stamina or physical ability as a person who only has a few pounds to drop. That's why the exercise program also varies according to your existing weight.

The three parts—the food plan, the physical exercises, and the mental exercises—all work together. If you skip the exercises, forget it. If you don't learn to have control over your mind, which eventually leads to controlling your appetite, this program is a waste of your time. The *teamwork* is what makes this way of losing weight, gaining energy, and having a better body unique. Now before you start, stop and think for a minute. How many pounds overweight are you?

Right now, without this book in your hands—how many pounds too much are you?

I know this is painful, so get it over quick. Just spit it out, write it on a piece of paper, and throw it away, if it hurts that much. Whatever the amount is, round the number off (if you are seventeen pounds over, just say twenty), find the program designed for you, and begin now! The longer you wait, the more weight you will accumulate, so do yourself a big favor and begin Living It.

As your weight changes, your Live-It Program will change, too. What you eat and the amount of exercise you have to do will vary as you progress from one plan to the next. Then when you are at your desired weight, your eating habits and exercise habits should be set for life. You will *always* have to exercise and to watch what you eat. But you will not always be overweight.

TOO MUCH VOLUME_____

One of the biggest problems with people on diets is that they firmly believe they're on a diet, when in reality they're eating way too much. They have faithfully forfeited Kentucky Fried Chicken and Big Macs, and are limiting themselves to health foods, yogurt and birdseed, but they aren't losing much weight and they don't know what the hell is wrong.

Volume is what's wrong. Too much volume—of anything but water—can do you in.

When I begin someone on the Live-It Program I ask them to fill in a chart of what they normally eat during a week. I ask for just the middle week days, because everyone cheats on the weekends. Before you make your own chart, take a look at one of the charts I got back from a woman who thought she was on a diet and couldn't understand why she wasn't losing weight.

TUESDAY
Breakfast
8:00 A.M.   1 slice of toast with margarine; 2 eggs, scrambled; glass of orange juice; 2 cups of coffee (milk, 2 sugars)

Snack
10:30 A.M.   Cup of peach yogurt

Lunch
12:30 P.M.   ½ turkey salad sandwich; 2 slices of fresh pineapple; glass of milk

Dinner
8:30 P.M.   Small salad; breast of barbecued chicken; one ear of corn with butter, salt; one glass of white wine; cup of coffee; ½ dinner roll

WEDNESDAY
Breakfast
8:00 A.M.   1 small glass of tropical fruit drink; 1 tablespoon of cottage cheese; piece of toast with margarine; 1 coffee (milk, 2 sugars)

Snack
10:30 A.M.   Handful of cherries

Lunch
1:00 P.M.   Spinach salad (with bacon bits, eggs, mushrooms, and vinaigrette dressing); 2 crackers; glass of milk

Dinner
9:00 P.M.   Seafood combination plate (fish, shrimp, scallops, fried in a batter—I remove the batter—I never liked that shit anyway); 4 french fries; 1 glass iced tea; 1 coffee (black)

Snack
10:30 P.M.   1 cookie (Oreo); 1 glass of warm milk

THURSDAY

Breakfast

8:00 A.M.   Glass of juice (tomato); ½ of spinach, onion, ground beef, and mushroom omelette; wedge of watermelon; 1 cup coffee (black)

Lunch

12:30 P.M.   Small dish of Jello-O; 1 bread stick; 1 diet drink

Dinner

9:00 P.M.   Tuna sandwich; ½ cantaloupe with fresh strawberries; 1 glass of water; 1 cup coffee (black)

Snack

10:30 P.M.   ½ cup strawberry yogurt

It doesn't take a degree in medicine or nutrition to figure out why Lady X hasn't lost any weight, now does it?

Although her choices were often sensible, her intake was equal to that of the Chinese Red Army. If you're eating sensible foods and gaining weight, maybe it's not the quality of the food but the quantity. Think about that while you fill in your own mid-week food chart, and then analyze the results. If you cheat here, you're only cheating yourself. . . .

Your Personal Mid-Week Food Chart___

TUESDAY
Breakfast

_____

_____

_____

_____

_____

_____

Lunch

_____

_____

_____

_____

_____

Dinner

_____

_____

_____

_____

_____

_____

_____

Snack

_____

_____

_____

_____

_____

WEDNESDAY
Breakfast

_____

_____

_____

_____

_____

Lunch

_____
_____
_____
_____

Dinner

_____
_____
_____
_____

Snack

_____
_____
_____

Dinner

_____
_____
_____

Snack

_____
_____
_____
_____
_____
_____

THURSDAY

Breakfast

_____
_____
_____
_____
_____

Lunch

_____
_____
_____

FOOD HARMONY

Many people, especially fat ones, eat what they want to eat when they feel like it. They never take into consideration what foods work for or against their bodies, or whether the intake from one meal balances with the previous meal.

To have a healthy body—and a thin one—you need to eat a proper balance of foods that will keep you in perfect harmony. After all, it's not nice to fool Mother Nature. Food has been broken down into four major food groups: Milk, Protein, Vegetable/Fruit, and Bread/Cereal. If you are putting away too much cheese, if a lot of pumpernickel is finding its way into your mouth, or if you eat enough fruit salad for two (because it's so healthy), then you are in big trouble.

Probably two sizes too big.

On the other hand, if you are not getting enough vegetables or protein you are also in trouble. The key word to it all is *balance*. Most people simply have not figured out how to balance their food intake. Food balance is very personal; what I can eat and function properly on may not be the same for you.

So how do you find the perfect balance for your body? By strictly following your Live-It Program and by paying attention, keeping tuned in to what you are eating, and adjusting your appetite to your body's needs. As you lose weight on the Live-It Program and move through the three body-type groupings, you will see your food harmony changing and adjusting to the new, thinner you. Watch for the signs your body gives you of change—they mean success.

An important factor in achieving proper food harmony in your body will be timing. The later in the day you eat, the lighter you must eat. During the day you have a chance to burn off heavier foods. At night you are less active. (If you have to sneak a snack, do it during daytime—not at night—especially not at bedtime.) Food harmony is built into your Live-It Program.

The Live-It Food Program, as well as the Exercise Program, is broken into three parts, depending on how much weight you need to lose. Begin with the appropriate category and move on as you lose weight. (You clever thing, you.)

THE LIVE-IT FOOD PROGRAM

Breakfast

Don't skip it. Sure, you'll lose weight faster if you don't eat the healthy necessities charted out for you, but your body won't function properly and you'll be in a rotten mood by noon. Get in the habit of making some time in the morning for the most important meal of the day.

Earlier in the book I told you about a drink I begin my mornings with:

> 8 oz. warm water
> the juice of a freshly squeezed lemon
> 1 teaspoon of honey

This drink is a suggestion, not a requirement, and does not appear on the food plan. If you have irregular bathroom habits and want to keep your insides spic and span, mix this drink and continue on to your meal.

Breakfast should not be eaten any later than 10:00 A.M. It just throws off the whole day if you eat after that hour, and your digestive system will have trouble gearing up for lunch.

Tips for Lunch

● Avoid soups made with a lot of cream and flour. Those "cream of whatever soups" aren't your best friends. Stick with soups made from stock, such as vegetable, chicken, etc. Who said anything about crackers? Not me. Just ignore them for now.

● I hate those diets that tell you to eat your salads with lemon juice or to ask for vinegar on the side. Ugh. Is that any way to live? Why don't you just order the house dressing—usually a vinaigrette—on the side and use just a teensy bit as you munch along? Or splurge on a dab of bleu cheese or Russian once a week—but only a dab.

● When ordering lunch, try to keep in mind what you just put in your stomach for breakfast. If you had eggs, don't order an open-face egg-salad sandwich. You don't need that many yolks! How about some sliced chicken on a slice of rye bread? Keep remembering not to duplicate the same food over and over again. The variety will keep you away from getting bored and tired of certain foods.

• Under beverage you notice that regular or sugar-free soft drinks are permitted at times. We are not counting calories or carbs on this plan. You make the choice as to whether you want to put a little more sugar or a few more artificial preservatives and synthetics in your body. These different drinks will not upset or unbalance your Live-It Program.

Dinner

More weight damage is done at dinner than at any other meal. Why? Well, there're several reasons. One is timing—which we've already talked about. Because you don't do too much later in the day, especially after you've eaten dinner, that big meal you've just eaten has no place to go but your hips. If you went out and boogied for five hours after eating it would be one thing—but not many people do that, and those who do don't keep it up every single night. To keep dinner in balance with the body one must remember this cardinal rule: the later the hour the lighter the meal. Got it?

Another problem with evenings is exhaustion. You've had a hard day at the office or with the kids or doing your thing and you're tired. You want a reward for making it through one more grueling day; you want a nice treat to ease over your tired body and perk you up. A meal without restrictions is what you assume will make you happy. But you're wrong. No matter how tired you are, or how much you think you deserve a break today, a light meal is important.

This isn't to say you should eat a carrot and a piece of parsley and call it a night, or that you can't sit around a table for hours and have a great time. It just means that you must watch your balance even more than ever. You can Live-It and still love nighttime eating.

PLAN A

Breakfast: If you have *fifty pounds or more to lose,* you have been naughty for a long, long time, haven't you? You've sort of given up on yourself and your body and only fantasize that you can be slimmer without really doing anything about it. That's going to stop right now. Sometimes you think no one cares? Well, I care. I mean, what if someone saw you carrying this book around and not losing any weight? That would make us both look pretty stupid—and personally, my ego just can't take that. Especially because I know this program works—and it works on extremely heavy people as well as it works on slightly pudgy people. So calm down and get with it. We're going to do this together. Take it slowly and easily—have a check-up by your doctor—and give yourself enough time to effect a healthy change in your body. Before you know it you'll be in Plan B. Until then, choose one from each column.

Lunch: If *fifty or more pounds* seem to be on your back, then you better back away from the lunches you are used to. You have convinced yourself that you'll eat a big lunch and forego dinner—but we know that seldom happens. You sometimes bring your lunch from home, eat it before noon, and end up going out with a business associate, just to keep him company, of course. You eventually keep company with a grilled cheese sandwich. Not too good. Try this plan instead. Choose one from each column.

Dinner: If you are *fifty or more pounds* over your desired weight the majority of those pounds were probably gained at dinnertime. You love to eat out, hate to do dishes. You take seconds too often, and it seems the bread and butter are always placed in front of you. Salt is one of your favorite things, and you hit the ketchup bottle pretty hard, too. By now all those fattening foods are starting to get boring. Your little taste buds are tired and ready for a change. Now's the time to wake them up with a good nutritious dinner. Choose one from each column.

Breakfast

A	B	C
Glass of juice	Hot or cold cereal (low-fat milk, honey, sugar, sugar substitute) (Only twice a week)	1 cup coffee, tea (as you like it)
or		
Piece of fruit	or	or
(papaya, orange, grapefruit—pineapple, grape, prune and apple only once a week)	2 eggs scrambled, poached (any way but fried) (only twice a week)	Low-fat milk (on days you don't have cereal)
or		Water (mineral or tap)
	or	
Sliced fruit (for cereal)	1 slice of toast with butter/margarine, or dab of jelly preserves, etc. (3 times a week)	
(sliced bananas only once a week)		

Lunch

A	B
Small salad*/small soup combo	Iced tea; hot coffee; tea (one cup or glass the way you like it)
Large vegetable salad with one protein included (cheese, turkey, chicken, etc.)	Water (mineral or tap)
Low-fat cottage cheese/fruit salad combo (once a week)	Soft drink (regular or sugar-free; allowed only twice a week)
Low-fat yogurt/fruit salad combo (once a week)	
Open-face sandwich (one piece of bread; meat must be lean; if tuna or egg salad, watch the mayo; once a week)	
*All dressings for salads must be served on side and used sparingly.	

Dinner

A	B	C	D
Small dinner salad (dressing on the side)	Portion of lean chicken (no skin) fish	Glass of wine with dinner twice a week	Iced tea; hot tea; coffee (one cup the way you like it)
One vegetable	or		Water (mineral or tap)
	(No liver, veal, lamb, lean red meat for now)		
	PLUS		
	1 baked potato (once a week or a half twice a week), dab of butter/margarine only		

Two evenings a week (your choice—I recommend two weekdays like Tuesday/Thursday) omit above Dinner Food Plan (A, B) and *ruffage it*. Make a large salad, including vegetables, plus one protein, dressing on side please. See *Salad Info*.

PLAN B

Breakfast: If you have *twenty to forty pounds to lose* you think it's only ten, and you've been kidding yourself and holding your stomach in for too long a time. You hate shopping for clothes with friends and get on a scale once a year around physical time, leaving the doctor's office very depressed. Your worries are over—at your next physical you'll even help the nurse weigh you in. Here's what you eat—one from each column, please.

Lunch: If you are *twenty to forty pounds too much* you go out too much for lunch and don't behave yourself. You love meeting a few friends at one of your favorite coffee-shops around the corner and you know the menu by heart. You drink too many glasses of water, and you just love to taste what others have ordered because you were afraid to order it yourself. Don't be afraid any more. Now you'll be able to have a tasty lunch—but watch how much water you're drinking, nobody can be that thirsty! Choose one from each column.

Dinner: If you have *twenty to forty pounds you'd like to see disappear,* you've come to the right place for dinner. You hate paper plates to eat off of and plastic utensils aren't your favorite either. You love appetizers like stuffed mushrooms, shrimp scampi, and Swedish meatballs—so who doesn't? You always order a dessert, saying "I know everyone will help me eat this ten-layered tart," but no one lifts a fork. You won't be having that tart for a while, but I plan to keep your fork busy and healthy. Choose one from each column.

Breakfast

A	B	C
Glass of juice	Hot or cold cereal (low-fat milk, honey, sugar, sugar substitute)	1 cup coffee, tea (as you like it)
or		
Piece of fruit	or	or
(pineapple, grape, prune and apple juice or fruit only twice a week)	2 eggs scrambled, poached (any way but fried)	Low-fat milk (on days you don't have cereal)
or	Plus 1 slice of toast, ½ muffin, etc. with butter/margarine *or* dab of jelly, preserves, etc. (Bread allowed only three times a week)	Water (mineral or tap)
Sliced fruit (when you have cereal)		
Limit sliced bananas to twice a week		

Lunch

A	B
Small salad*/small cup of soup combo	Iced tea; hot coffee; tea (one cup or glass the way you like it)
Large vegetable salad with one protein included (cheese, turkey, chicken, etc.)	Water (mineral or tap)
Low-fat cottage cheese/fruit salad combo	Soft drink (regular or sugar-free; allowed only four times a week)
Low-fat yogurt/fruit salad combo	
Open-face sandwich** (one piece of bread; meat must be lean; if tuna or egg salad, watch the mayo)	
*All dressings for salads must be served on side and used sparingly	
**Sandwich allowed only on days you don't have bread for breakfast	

Dinner

A	B	C	D
Small dinner salad (dressing on the side)	Portion of lean chicken (no skin), fish, or veal (portion of lamb, lean red meat, liver once a week)	Glass of wine with dinner four times a week	Iced tea; hot tea; coffee (one cup the way you like it)
Cup of soup (watch out for the creamy ones)	PLUS		Water (mineral or tap)
Small glass of tomato or V-8 juice	One vegetable (see *Veg. Info.*)		
	PLUS		
	1 baked potato (once a week or a half twice a week) dab of butter/margarine or sour cream		
	Brown rice (twice a week; (recipe to follow)		

Two evenings a week (your choice—I recommend two weekdays like Tuesday/Thursday) omit above dinner Food Plan (A,B) and *ruffage it*. Make a large salad, including vegetables, plus one protein, dressing on side, please. See *Salad Info*.

PLAN C

Breakfast: If you have *one to fifteen pounds to lose* you're probably in the worst category of dieter—you know you need to lose some weight but it's not so much for you to take it entirely seriously, so you go through life trying new diets, taking off a few pounds and never losing the full amount or keeping it off. You've been on every existing diet ever invented but are very fickle—you'll jump to whatever hot diet craze you hear about next, especially if you think your excess pounds will go away quickly, easily, and without too much work. Poor you—deluding yourself all these years. Well, now's your chance. With the Live-It Program you can take off all the weight, keep it off and see your body in better shape than it's ever been in since you were six. You just have to care about yourself enough to really do it. Choose one from each column, and enjoy.

Lunch: If you have *one to fifteen pounds to get rid of,* lunches are really not a problem for you since you normally don't eat lunch except for an apple that's been in your desk for a few days. You usually read on your lunch hour and chew a half a pack of sugarless gum. You may go out for lunch once a week and eat all the crust off the bread in the basket. It's time to add a little more zip to your life—and for God's sake, clean out your desk.

Dinner: If you are *one to fifteen pounds overweight,* by now you are pretty sick of water-packed tuna and have tried every damn diet frozen dinner on the market. You are beginning to believe that you will never lose those last few pounds and you're about to rush out and nibble on some grass. Before attacking your lawn, give this plan an honest try.

Breakfast

A	B	C
Glass of juice (any kind)	Hot or cold cereal (low-fat milk, honey, sugar, sugar substitute)	1 cup coffee, tea (as you like it)
or		or
Piece of fruit (any kind)	or	Low-fat milk (on days you don't have cereal)
or	2 eggs scrambled, poached (any way but fried)	Water (mineral or tap)
Sliced fruit (when you have cereal)	PLUS	
	1 slice of toast, ½ muffin, etc. with butter/margarine *or* jelly, preserves, etc.	

Lunch

A	B
Small salad*/small cup of soup combo	Iced tea; hot coffee or tea (one cup or glass the way you like it)
Large vegetable salad with one protein included (cheese, turkey, chicken, etc.)	Water (mineral or tap)
Low-fat cottage cheese/fruit salad combo	Soft drink (regular or sugar free)
Low-fat yogurt/fruit salad combo	
Open-face sandwich (one piece of bread; meat must be lean; if tuna or egg salad, watch the mayo.)	
*All dressings for salads must be served on side and used sparingly	

Dinner

A	B	C	D
Small dinner salad (dressing on side)	Portion of lean chicken (no skin), fish, or veal	1 glass of wine with dinner every night	Iced tea; hot tea; coffee (one cup or glass the way you like it)
Cup of soup (watch out for creamy ones)	(Portion of lamb, lean red meat, liver—twice a week)	or	Water (mineral or tap)
Small glass of tomato juice or V-8 juice	PLUS	1 alcoholic beverage with dinner 3 times a week	
	One vegetable (see *Veg. Info.*)	(That knocks out all the wine)	
	PLUS		
	1 baked potato (once a week or a half twice a week) dab of butter, margarine or sour cream		
	Brown rice (twice a week; recipe to follow)		

Two evenings a week (your choice—I recommend two weekdays like Tuesday/Thursday) omit above dinner Food Plan (A,B) and *ruffage it*. Make a large salad, including vegetables, plus one protein, dressing on side, please. See *Salad Info*.

TIPS AND RECIPES FOR DINNER

How to Fix Your Protein

Chicken

You can lightly season the chicken parts with pepper, parsley, paprika, dill, oregano, tarragon, or any other of your favorite spices, and bake or broil in the oven. No salt! Cook with the skin on to keep the meat moist and tender, but remove the skin before you devour Mr. Chicken. I know, you don't have to tell me the skin tastes wonderful, but it's pure fat—the exact thing we are trying to lose.

I can speak from experience that a piece of chicken thrown in the oven or barbequed can get pretty boring, so try this tasty dish:

10-Minute Chicken

• Debone and skin a few thighs or a breast; cut up in chunks and marinate in 3 tablespoons soy sauce or Worcestershire for a few minutes while preparing the rest of the ingredients.
• Slice up some carrots, zucchini, celery, onions (a small amount of each, which counts for your vegetable allowance).
• Get the Teflon pan out and turn burner on medium.
• Add 2 tablespoons water; sautée vegetables until they are semicooked.
• Now turn burner on high, add pieces of chicken (but not the remaining sauce), and keep tossing the mixture around till the chicken is cooked.

There are so many casserole combinations of chicken and vegetables in which butter and sauces aren't needed. Start experimenting!

Fish

Most people hate to cook fish at home because it smells up the kitchen and is sort of messy. If you marinate salmon, halibut, trout, sea bass, whatever, in lemon or lime juice for a few minutes and then bake or broil it the odor problem is eliminated and the fish will stay tender during cooking. Once in a while pick up some fresh shrimp, but only once in a while, till we see your eating habits improve. (No lobster—I'm afraid you'll be like me and go straight for the butter.)

You can prepare your choice of seafood just like the chunks of chicken (only marinate in soy sauce—Worcestershire and fish don't mix); this time by using bean sprouts and mushrooms as your vegetable allowance.

Veal

Veal gets tough very quickly. Whether you buy it sliced thin or in the form of a veal chop, you should broil or sautée it for only a few minutes. Dill or tarragon adds a nice touch to veal. Strips of veal can also be marinated like chicken for a veal and vegetable stew.

Liver

I eat calves' liver every Monday night. I take my Teflon pan, turn the burner on medium, and sautée sliced onions in four tablespoons of water. I add fresh-ground pepper and parsley and cook till the onions begin browning—no butter or oil is necessary. I then place a few small wafer-thin slices of liver in the same pan, and in four minutes dinner is ready. Chicken livers are a bit more fatty, and if you're not a liver lover, calves' liver is more pleasant.

Steak

Red meat has been knocked around for the last couple of years, but it hasn't stopped too many people from cutting into a good sirloin occasionally. Steak can be sautéed in the Teflon pan also, and marinated in the two sauces I mentioned. There's nothing wrong with steak and vegetables on allowed days. Just make sure you cut off all the visible fat. If you're in the mood for a hamburger patty, buy the chuck and have it ground right in front of you. Most hamburger meat for sale already packed has a high fat content, which you're trying to avoid.

Protein is a very necessary requirement for your Live-It Program. Most of us have been introduced to meat, fish, and fowl accompanied with gravies, mystery sauces, and batter. Now's the time to enjoy the real taste of chicken or Mahi-Mahi without the fattening extras.

Potatoes and Rice

Can I Have a Potato?

In my heavier days I could make one or two baked potatoes, "with everything," disappear in no time. Then potatoes went through some bad publicity and people suddenly threw them right out of their lives. Sure, french fries, hash browns, and potato pancakes are very little potato and a lot of grease, and if you look around and watch others eat their goodies, you'll always see a salt shaker and bottle of ketchup close by.

But the potato itself has a lot of pros in the vitamin department and that's why most of you are allowed a taste. Here's what I do: I cut the potato in half and wrap just one half in tinfoil and bake. When it's ready I add a bit of butter/margarine, just a bit, some pepper, and fresh chopped chives.

The half is very filling, and you have the other half in the fridge for when the potato mood strikes again. Don't forget to scrub the skin and eat every bit of it.

Brown Rice

Buy the short-grain brand. Get out a heavy pan with a lid that closes tightly. First:

● Chop up a little bit of celery and onions, sautée in water, and add a pinch of thyme or any of your favorite herbs.
● Throw in 1 cup raw rice, turn heat up, and sautée rice and vegetable mixture for a few minutes. Add 2 cups cold water and bring to a boil.
● Turn heat on low and cook for 1 hour. Cover and don't touch the pan or lift the lid.

This recipe can be made days earlier and kept in the fridge. When you're ready to eat, just heat up a portion in a few tablespoons of water and enjoy.

How to Prepare Vegetables

If you take my suggestion and mix your protein with a few vegies, please remember that counts for your vegetable allowance. On the days you are content with a few slices of turkey (that's just a bigger chicken) or a nice piece of filet of sole, you must begin learning the art of cooking vegetables. Now just look how most restaurants treat string beans and carrots—boil them till there's not a vitamin left, then drench them in butter or some other kind of sauce. I personally could eat leaves if they had a butter sauce on top of them.

Here're a few tips:
● Invest in a steamer and steam the vegetables until they're crisp. Zucchini, celery,

squash, onions, and those tiny Italian tomatoes take about 6 minutes to cook after the water starts to boil. Carrots, cauliflower, broccoli, asparagus, and a few of the harder vegies take a little longer—12 to 15 minutes. Corn is America's #1 choice for a vegetable, but by the time you finish buttering, salting, and peppering that cob, it's also America's #1 vegetable that's the most fattening, so be careful.

• Eating only one vegetable a night is very unimaginative. Slice up some zucchini, add a few mushrooms, some carrots and peas, and place them in the steamer (remember which vegetables take the longest to cook—those go in first), sprinkle with basil and some chopped garlic, and you've just created a healthy, nonfattening dish. If you're not in the meat, fish, or fowl mood one evening, there's nothing wrong with a portion of that brown rice and a nice vegetable casserole.

• Besides steaming vegetables (please don't say the word "boil" around vegies), use the Teflon pan again or a wok to prepare very crispy vegetables. Add 1 tablespoon oil and 1 tablespoon soy sauce to the pan, which should be on high heat. Throw the vegetables in and toss around constantly. The other night I sliced up fresh asparagus and broccoli, sautéed them for 4 minutes, then added snow peas, parsley, and onions. Look through some cookbooks and get some ideas about which vegetables taste good with which.

• Certain vegetables are unbelievable when baked. Fresh beets, squash, baked cabbage with rye seeds taste terrific. You wrap them in foil, season, and stick them in the oven. The water content from the vegetables manufactures a natural juice, so who needs all that butter?

◇ ◇ ◇

Lean Is Green

By now you've noticed that I have a tender spot in my heart for salads. Remember I mentioned earlier special foods that could make you healthy, wealthy, and wise? Well, they're all in the salads I plan to teach you about. Eating salads the required two nights or more on your food plan is the real secret to dropping excess weight and keeping your health in order. Anything you can put between bread or cover with gravy can be mixed together with greens, and there're so many kinds of salads to prepare that you'll never get tired of them.

Whether you are having a small salad with dinner or plan to feast on a salad as your main meal, it doesn't matter. Many of the vegetables you steamed and weren't able to finish should be placed in the fridge and used in a salad the next evening. Certain people have a tender tummy and many raw vegetables cause them digestion problems.

Here are a few salad suggestions:

• It seems the whole world uses iceberg lettuce as a salad base. Spend more time in the produce section and pick up some other lettuce, such as Romaine, endive, butter lettuce. Thinly sliced red or green cabbage can be substituted if you desire a different taste.

• Many vegetables can be marinated and then added to the salad. Steamed string beans, beets (it's O.K. to boil these), tomatoes, yellow squash can soak in a little vinaigrette dressing for added flavor. Marinated cucumber and onions is a salad in itself.

• When making the salad don't forget not to duplicate your proteins. If you had eggs for breakfast and turkey for lunch, add some tuna to your evening greeneries. If you were on good behavior all day, a chef's salad once in a while is perfect. A few slices of cheese, julienne strips of chicken, and a couple slivers of roast beef lying on a bed of lettuce with tomatoes, radishes, green peas, mushrooms, and onions. What a masterpiece!

• Before you become a big fan of salads, you must develop some patience for washing, peeling, chopping, and slicing. Good salads take a little more time, but it's worth it. You must make sure that the vegetables are very clean—they are mostly grown in dirt, you know. Also, make sure all the lettuce leaves and various vegies are dried off after washing before you add dressing.

• Speaking of dressings—here's the fatty problem that usually ruins the reputation of healthy salads. Dressings are to salads as gravy is to mashed potatoes. No one is asking you to eat your bowl of greens dry, but no one's asking you to finish off a bowl of dressing, either. That's why the tablespoon was invented, so you can spoon on a moderate amount of your favorite dressing. Every vegetable in your salad doesn't have to be covered with blue cheese or Russian dressing. Always order your dressing on the side and again, remember not to duplicate your food groups. On the days you've had your dairy allowance, choose a dressing free of yogurt, mayo, or half and half. Pick an Italian dressing or an oil-based one.

• Also watch out for salad toppings. Croutons, sunflower seeds, Parmesan cheese, garbanzo beans, etc. can add pounds to your hips in no time. If you need a few croutons

or whatever to decorate the top of your salad choose to do so at lunch, but not at the last meal of the day.

Here are a few salad-dressing recipes you might want to try out. Remember, don't take a bath in them, learn to use that spoon. A little dab will do you.

Buttermilk Dressing
1 cup buttermilk
¼ cup cottage cheese (low-fat)
1 tablespoon mayonnaise
1 tablespoon dill
½ teaspoon ground pepper
Add: (minced finely)
        1 small bunch parsley
        ¼ cup bell pepper
        ¼ cup yellow onion
Mix together well and chill.

Tomato Vinaigrette
½ cup tomato juice
¼ cup apple cider vinegar
¼ cup lemon juice (fresh)
¼ cup cottonseed oil (or pure vegetable oil)
1 teaspoon thyme
1 teaspoon garlic
1 teaspoon ground pepper
Sprinkle sea salt (optional)

Blend and store in the fridge.
Now, in Cuisinart (or any food processor, or chopped by hand) chop fine:1 small bunch of parsley
1 bunch green onions (5 or 6)

Add above to what's in the fridge and you've got yourself a zesty vinaigrette dressing that can also be used to marinate meats and/or vegetables.

Yogurt Garlic Dressing
1 cup low-fat plain yogurt
1 teaspoon fresh lime juice
1 minced clove garlic
2 tablespoons parsley, chopped
1 tablespoon chives, chopped
½ teaspoon ground pepper
Put all ingredients in a bowl and blend well with a whisk.

Here's an easy vegetable soup I've been serving in my restaurant for four years and nobody's tired of it.

Ruffage Vegetable Soup
1 can tomato juice (24 oz.)
1 teaspoon ground pepper
1 teaspoon oregano
1 shake of sea salt
Bring above to a boil. Throw in 4 cups of the following vegetables:
cubed tomatoes
chopped bell pepper
chopped onions
shredded cabbage
sliced celery
sliced carrots
sliced zucchini
sliced mushrooms
bean sprouts
Cover, lower heat, and simmer till vegetables are cooked but crisp.

MAINTAINING YOUR WEIGHT

One of the most depressing things about a diet has always been the fact that soon after you've taken off the weight you almost killed yourself taking off, you gain it back. You usually end up right where you began, prediet, or even heavier. It's frustrating, upsetting, irritating, and also unhealthy.

You will keep off all the weight you lost with the Live-It Program because it is not a crash diet. My program has been designed to last a lifetime. Once you get to your desired weight, all you need to do is stay on the Live-It Maintenance Program and you'll live happily ever after—without, I might add, ever having to read another diet book in your life.

As we've already noted several times, the Live-It Program is a three-pronged process combining exercise, mental attitudes, and a food plan. On the maintenance program you will continue the steady combination of these three vital programs.

The Live-It Maintenance Program is your insurance policy. Read and reread it. Every day, if you have to. Memorize it. Let it become your Bible. You've made it this far (have I told you how proud I am?) and I want you to go all the way—to keep the weight off for the rest of your life. To do this you must accept the basic tenets of the Live-It Program: exercise and controlled eating are always going to be part of your life. You cannot revert to your former self and expect to keep the weight off. You can't pick up one of those has-been excuses, like "I don't feel well today, I'll just sit this one out," or "I deserve to eat this" every day and expect to remain as slender as a model. You must be in control of your life and your habits or you will regain, not maintain.

This is not to say that you will spend the rest of your life going from Column A to Column B and never once eating a piece of pizza or a deep-dish apple pie with cinnamon and raisins. What I think is so great about the Live-It Maintenance Program is that it allows you to eat anything you want.

You heard me—*anything you want*—who can forget ice cream or chocolate? Or beer-batter fried shrimp with tartar sauce or hot homemade bread straight from the oven with warm jam and butter? Other diets will tell you never to think about these foods again. I say that you're only human and you have to live like a person.

So, if you want a waffle with everything on it for breakfast, go ahead, have it. But not every morning. One day a week will suffice, thank you. And make sure that on the same day you have the waffle you don't have a club sandwich, double order of fries, half a box of chocolate cookies, and a few beers.

You will never again be able to eat the way you ate before you began the diet. But do you really want to? You can have anything you may ever want—you just can't have it all at once, and you would do well not to finish it.

The trick to the Live-It Maintenance Program is to alternate the food program for the lowest weight loss (Food Plan C) with a normal life-style diet of your favorite healthy foods. That is to say, if you have the waffle we just mentioned for breakfast on Sunday, you must follow the Food Plan C for the rest of the day. On Monday, you should have breakfast from Food Plan C, but you can alternate lunch or dinner with the selection of your choice.

This doesn't mean you can pig-out at one meal each day, because you probably can't. It means that you can pig-out with moderation once a week as long as you control the rest of your weekly diet. Exercise, sometimes extra exercise, will combat an oink-oink session, and fasting may be necessary the day immediately following an all-out splurge.

But all your mistakes are correctable. You can quickly and quietly get yourself out of any overweight mess you get yourself into before it's too late and you've gone, shall we say, whole hog.

One of the checks and balances of this system of correcting boo-boos is to weigh yourself every day. Never cringe at the thought of facing your old enemy the scale. If you've come this far you have beaten Mr. Scale and you should be proud to toe the line once a day. It's normal for weight to fluctuate slightly—your menstrual cycle, a change of weather, irregular bathroom habits can alter your regular weight by two to three pounds, so you should always give yourself a two- to-three pound leeway. Any more than that, don't blame Mother Nature or a broken scale.

Now don't get neurotic about weighing yourself and rush onto the scale two or three times a day or after every meal. Once a day will do it but at the same time every day, please.

Believe me, the easiest way in the world of maintaining your weight is by weighing every day. If you miss just one day, a pound may creep up. If you miss a few days, it could be a few pounds creeping. Don't take the chance. Why gamble? Weigh yourself once a day and stay in control.

Now then, if you notice a change in your weight—say of one or two pounds—that is your warning signal. It may be Mother Nature, it may be the chocolate-mousse pie you ate last night. Be very careful that day—exercise a little bit more strenuously and watch your food intake meticulously. If the weight has not fallen off the next day it's time for action: Revert to strict use of Food Plan C for the next three days. Exercise with care and a little more enthusiasm. Check your mental attitude and give yourself the necessary pep talks to stay in control and beat back the pounds before they capture your soul.

You must also understand that you will be exercising for the rest of your life. You must make certain that all your blood circulates properly and that your body remains limber, flexible, and firm—whether you're fifteen, fifty, or one hundred fifteen. If you stop and start your exercise program you are stopping and starting your life. Don't fall into that trap. *You are never finished* taking care of yourself, and that's as it should be.

The scale is your checkpoint. The mirror is your witness. Your mind must serve as guardian angel. Your mental attitude is the third and an equally important part of your weight-loss and maintenance program. Don't ignore it.

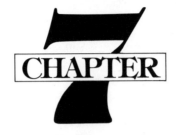

CHAPTER 7

YOUR MENTAL ATTITUDE: YOUR GUARDIAN ANGEL

INTRODUCTION

I've always found that my mental attitude is directly related to my appearance. When I was fat, I often hated myself, was unhappy, and had to eat to make myself feel better. It was that awful cycle we've all endured, and it seemed there was no way to break out of it.

Yet it was a mental process which made me first grab hold of myself to lose weight, and several other mental attitudes which reinforced me throughout the ordeal of weight loss and the difficulties of maintenance. And finally it was mental attitude that changed my life when I realized that it was no longer hard to remain thin, that I no longer thought of maintenance as maintenance but

as my regular life plan and that I knew that I would never be fat again.

If the cliché makers can tell you that mind triumphs over matter, I also suggest that mind can triumph over fatter. The very first step in beginning to lose weight is the acknowledgment that "you can do it."

Once I said those four words I needed a little backup reinforcement, but I was on my way. There have been days of my life that I have not been able to get out of bed without mentally whipping myself into shape and assuring myself that whatever it was, "I could do it." This attitude will be essential in your successful weight loss.

But you don't just say "I can do it" once, the day you buy this book, and never think about it again. You must do what I had to do for myself . . . give yourself an entire set of mental exercises and attitudes to carry you through the weight-loss and maintenance program. It's like whistling a happy tune—you'll fool yourself as well as others when you adapt an attitude that gives no way for defeat.

YOU HAVE IT IN YOU TO BE THIN

What made you buy this book in the first place? What made you tackle all those other miserable diets and suffer through them with such ferocity? Your mind did. That little voice inside your being that knew you didn't want to be overweight any more and prodded you along the route to self-improvement. We all have a guardian angel inside ourselves; we just all don't listen.

An important part of the Live-It Program involves not only listening to that little voice but helping it to develop into an authority on your well-being and a force in your life that will help you keep in line. Your angel may just whisper or he may have to shout, that depends on you, but your body must obey.

You may have what it takes to be President of the United States or a movie star or a cheerleader, or anything else you want to be. You do have it in you to be thin and healthy for the rest of your life. And that's not something to take lightly.

As you study this book, and the Live-It Program, you should come to see how the bad eating habits and excuses of your past have put you where you are now and how your regular eating habits differ from the Live-It Program. You can reconcile these differences by retraining your guardian angel.

Only you can train yourself to begin new eating habits. Only you can listen to the voice that will say, "Have a salad today instead of a Big Mac." And unless you are able to pattern your subconscious into accepting a healthy new life-style, you will never correct your old eating patterns and will never take off enough weight to matter.

How do you make these changes? By exercising your mind just as you would your body.

THE LIVE-IT MENTAL-EXERCISE PROGRAM

Your mind comprehends habits through repetition. The more you think something or do something over and over again, the more these things shape your personality and style—good and bad. All the exercises I'm about to teach you are based on positiveness. I do these exercises every day without fail.

If you too will practice these exercises repeatedly, your mind will help guide you through any food crisis, and you'll end up a winner. If you quit, start skipping days, you will lose—your bad eating habits will never be replaced by good ones, the excess weight will always be around, and you'll feel uncomfortable the rest of your life. Please take my advice—study these mental exercises and put them into practice. They work. You won't believe how sharp your mind will become.

Positive-Suggestion Exercises

When you get up in the morning, right before you begin doing your physical exercises, head for the bathroom, look in the mirror, and say,

"Today I'm going to do better."

"I'm going to be in a very up, positive mood.'

"I'm going to succeed."

The above statements are not commands or demands. You don't have to threaten yourself anymore. Threats are negative tactics you've used in the past, and they don't work. You simply have to plant daily positive thoughts in the conscious part of your mind. Wherever you go, you are with you. You shouldn't worry about someone else and how he got the weight off. You don't go home with his body—you have to go home with yours.

The decisions about doing "better" have to be *your* decisions. Sure, you have friends who try to help you lose weight by making remarks like "You shouldn't be eating that" or "You're not supposed to be snacking," but those remarks are offensive to you unless you are ready in your mind to accept help from others.

You must be a good salesman to train yourself at that morning mirror. You have to look straight into your eyes and be convincing. Then and only then will those positive suggestions start taking over the negative patterns in your subconscious.

The Want-Need Exercises

All day long you are faced with decisions—and many of these have to do with food. Instead of just opening your mouth, start opening your mind by questioning yourself and then evaluating your answers.

Example:

It's a few hours after dinner. You had a good balanced dinner. You left the table satisfied, but for whatever reason (boredom, depression, loneliness) you feel like eating something.

Question Period:

"Do I *want* this?" "Yes, I want this chicken leg. Just this one time. I feel like eating, that's all. I know I'm spoiled and I shouldn't have it, but I won't do it again."

"Do I *need* this?" "No, I really don't need to eat a thing. I mean, it's almost bedtime. My body sure doesn't need any more food to digest—my dinner is still digesting. What I really need is to have self-control and stay on my food program. Anyway, if I were to give in and eat that drumstick, I'd have to go through a guilt trip ten minutes later."

The *needs* definitely override the *wants*, wouldn't you agree? Since in the past you never questioned your mind, you simply ate whatever you wanted and faced the fat later. Now you must start letting your mind be the judge. So no matter where you are or who you're with, stare at that food the way you stared at yourself in the mirror that morning. "Do I need this or do I want this?" This exercise strengthens your mental awareness. No longer does food and eating become mechanical—*you* are now in charge. You are reintroducing food to your body for a reason now, instead of through an excuse.

Mind-Signal Exercises

When I see the number 13, a black cat, or a ladder, I avoid them. When I'm in the market and I see apples, I always think to myself, "An apple a day keeps the doctor away." The peace symbol, a cross, the McDonald arch, a red light—we all know what they mean instantly when we see them. The magic of certain objects, words, and phrases can be very helpful to use when following this food program. Again, you are training your mind, thus constructing positive eating patterns.

Here're a few that I've repeatedly used for years. When I now hear certain words/phrases or see certain objects, they set off red lights and warning signals in my mind and I am able to deal with temptations objectively.

"I know you're watching your weight, but just take a *sliver* of this." The signal word is *sliver;* when you hear this word think, "A sliver leads to a slab, a slab leads to a slob." Right now you are not a one-bite eater; you may not be able to handle just a sliver of something. Little tastes lead to bigger tastes, which you don't need. So you begin associating words to results you aren't interested in. Sliver = slobs; tiny = ton; a bite = bloat. There are hundreds of these you can use to control your mind and appetite.

There are so many visual warnings when you eat out! Picking up the menu or lifting the basket of bread and noticing how heavy it is can keep you on your food program. Maybe your waiter or waitress is overweight. Maybe someone at the next table is gorging himself. I mean these should do something to make you order with caution and not go crazy over a meal that could keep you from your goals.

My favorite visual warning, which works whether I'm alone or in a room filled with people and food, is picking up the *fork.* When I pick up a fork, I quickly turn the fork so I see its profile. Do you know that a fork has about the thinnest profile I've ever seen? And that thin profile just digs into all that food and the results are anything but thin! Matter of fact, they're on the wide side. Try this one at your next meal. Get that fork in your hand, turn it to profile, let

your mind take a picture of that. Certain images will start filling your head. The fork is like a crane shovel digging in piles of food and dropping all that food in the ol' mouth. Whichever images work for you and keep you from pigging out are the ones you should use.

*End-of-the-Day Exercise*_____

Just as you began your day with a little positive pep talk, so should you end your day with some comforting words before doing your evening exercises. Look in that mirror one more time. Go through your day while it's fresh in your memory. Did you eat the right foods on your program? Did you do your morning exercises? Did you get angry and flunk out a few times? All right, be able to discuss those bad times with yourself. No one is perfect every day. Come on, don't pout or give up on me—or you. Look in that mirror and say to yourself;

"I will be realistic in my goals."

"The weight is not going to come off overnight, but it will come off."

"I must be patient and keep trying."

"Tomorrow will be a better day."

With confrontations like these, morning and evening—every day—you are reinforcing the self-love and respect you should have for yourself. Your mind will start rejecting all the habit patterns that make you feel rejected. Your mental exercises are the key to your Live-It Program.

STARTING NOW_____

You begin your mental-attitude program today, as you finish this book. (There's only one more chapter; don't quit now.) Here's what you do next.

• Get a pen, a magic marker, or one of those cute underlining yellow markers whose color you can see through as you draw through the words on a page. Don't use a pencil if you can help it.

• With pen in hand, begin this book again. This time you'll skim, marking the areas that particularly pertain to your case. Excuses that you know you've used before; areas of weakness that deep inside you can admit to; old familiar tales and sore points that apply to you personally. It shouldn't take much more than an hour or two to do this, and it's very important. The marked areas of the book are your own personal clues to where you will need the most reinforcement mentally and where you will have to retrain yourself and your living patterns to perfect your life-style.

• Memorize or list your weak points as outlined in the book; admit to them and accept them.

• Develop a personal set of mental exercises, based on repetition at the beginning, that will help you to transcend these weak areas. Train yourself to have your guardian angel give your body a new message when you're in one of the trouble situations. If you recognize that you hate exercise and will think of any old excuse to squirm out of it, then begin to train yourself to accept and then appreciate exercise and what it will do for you. You must repattern your bad habits, or you'll be sunk.

• As you work on each habit that has to be rebuilt and tackle your food and exercise programs, remind yourself constantly, "I CAN DO IT."

• I did it. And I know you can do it, too!

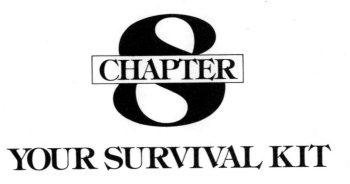

YOUR SURVIVAL KIT

INTRODUCTION

We've taken a tour of your past and your present. We've read about some things you've already known and some things you haven't thought about in a long time. But we're not through yet. You must protect your future.

You should now be ready to tackle your weight problem and come out the victor. You read this book to help you change your life forever. Now you should be ready to start that change.

There are just a few other things you should know. Remember at the beginning of the book when I told you about my own overweight problems? Remember the hair I lost that didn't grow back? Well, I had to have six hair-transplant operations. (Ouch!) I lost all my weight in such a hurry (over a hundred pounds in two and a half months— wouldn't you call that a hurry?). And needless to say, I got real skinny and I got real sick. First my face fell in! There was skin hanging everywhere—I looked like a newborn bald ostrich. At the age of nineteen I had to have a face lift. There were so many bags around my eyes that I looked like a luggage salesman, so I had my eyes done. In fact, when you look at the face on the cover of this book, you are looking at the approximate cost of a 1980 fully equipped Cadillac.

All this happened because I was so stupid and made enough mistakes for all of us.

This is not to say you might not want to

make some cosmetic changes when you're all through. A new hairstyle, maybe a new hair color. Maybe more. I know one woman who lost sixty pounds and celebrated by having her now sagging bosoms reduced to a smaller and tighter version of the same. It may take some getting used to the new you, so don't panic after you lose the pounds. When anyone in my classes loses the desired amount of weight, I go with her to the cosmetic department of a nearby store and show her how to redesign her face. I've taken people shopping for new clothes, hoping it will give them the incentive to stay thin and healthy forever.

Besides a little cosmetic lift, you are going to need those mental exercises to help you every step of the way. The rest of this chapter is designed for your use today and forever . . . to help you get that weight off and keep that weight off.

Oh yes, there's something very important you should know. This book comes with a ghost. That's right. It's haunted by me. I plan to haunt you every place you go, until your excess weight disappears . . . until you have respect for your body and until you learn how to have a good time no matter where you go and what you eat . . . or don't eat.

All right, get your scissors ready and your Scotch tape. I want you to cut out these graphs, lists, and illustrations and put them in their appropriate places. You never know when I will be coming to your house for inspection.

Oh yes—there's one more thing before you go on: burn all your old pictures. If you refuse to burn them, hide them. Yesterday is gone, my friend; those were the fat days. Today is the first day of the rest of your new slim life.

These are the first X-fat-rated illustrations ever published. Sexy, aren't they? I dare you to eat something fattening while staring at these pictures. Now are you convinced that FAT AIN'T BEAUTIFUL?

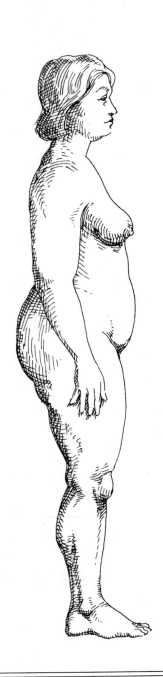

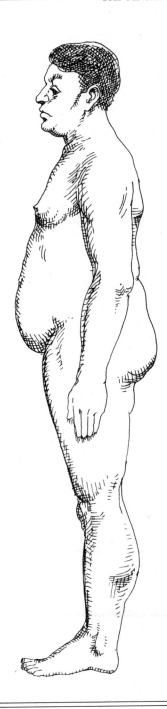

Medical Checklist

You may have had some bad experiences with doctors who weren't able to help you send your baby fat away. Now that you have this book you can afford to be generous. Forgive them and forget about them. But you're going to need a good doctor, so find someone you are happy with and make sure that everything in your body is in working order.

Before you begin any major weight-loss program, check with that doctor. Tell him what you are planning to do. Make sure you have no hidden complications and are fully aware of the areas you will need to go slower in when it comes to exercise.

My ideas have been practiced by thousands of people and checked over by several medical doctors. Nothing I have recommended to you will harm you. I may tire you out. You may curse and hate me, but it's all medically sound advice. But you can overdo it, and you should be aware of your physical condition before you begin.

1. Have a complete physical once a year and a checkup before you begin this exercise and weight-reduction plan.
2. Call your dentist for your six months' checkup, you're overdue. His phone number is ———/——— .
3. Make an appointment for a thorough eye examination, which should be followed up every year whether you wear glasses or not.
4. (Ladies) Learn breast self-examination techniques and practice them monthly after your menstrual cycle. Also have a regular gynecological examination and Pap smear.
5. Try to quit smoking. (I refuse to beg.)
6. If something hurts and doesn't go away within twenty-four hours get on the phone and call your doctor. Don't just lie there in pain and expect it to go away.
7. Make sure every member of your family follows the same medical checklist.

Cut this out and tape it inside your clothes closet.

Bathroom Chart

1. Keep your skin clean. Find a soap or cream and a rinse for the face that you believe in and use them morning and evening. You may have a thinner face now, so there's no excuse for a dirty one.

2. Keep those teeth clean. Brush them, floss them, Water-Pik them, gargle, and please brush your tongue. That's right, I said your tongue. All that food clogs your taste buds, and bad breath is often caused by a clogged-up tongue.

3. Keep your hair clean. Keep it conditioned. Don't put off regular visits to have it cut or styled.

4. Take better care of your hands and feet. There is something called a manicure. There is no reason to eat foods that will help strengthen your nails if you don't plan to take care of them.

5. Use a deodorant. I don't want you to receive anonymous surprise packages that contain a leading brand of antiperspirant (how embarrassing!).

6. Please leave your pimples alone. Do not pop them. They are nature's way of telling you something's wrong. Let them heal all by themselves and prevent the scars often caused by squeezing.

7. If you can't hear so well—I said, If you can't hear so well—maybe you have a wax build-up in your ears. Keep them clean.

8. Aside from keeping your skin clean, keep it moisturized. There is nothing attractive about dry, flaky, scaly skin. Use a good moisturizer daily from head to toe.

9. Shower in the mornings to wake you up and bathe in the evenings to relax you. Remember not real hot water. It not only makes the bills higher but also your body temperature.

10. Weigh yourself every day. I don't care if you decide to get on that scale in the morning or in the evening, but get on it. This constant checking will keep you aware of your progress.

Cut this chart out and tape it to the inside of your medicine cabinet. (If your medicine cabinet is not clean, I recommend you to get it in spic-and-span shape before I ring your doorbell.)

Outside-Refrigerator Chart

This works a lot better than a pretty picture taped to your refrigerator door. No, it's not a list of things to eat or not to eat. It's just a friendly little speech that your refrigerator would make—if it knew how to talk.

● Hi! No, nothing's new.
● What do you really want in here?
● I already told you there's nothing new since the last time you opened me.
● By the way, I can't remember the last time you cleaned me out. That jar of strawberry jam has got to go, and about the third shelf—not good. Not good at all. If you don't get at me with a little Ajax and warm water I might just faint from whatever is go-ing on in the third shelf.
● What? Back again? And without the Ajax? You already ate breakfast! How dare you come back so soon!
● Pardon me, but you're fondling my left-overs and I don't like it a bit. Now close this door and get the hell out of here. The left-overs are for dinner tonight!
● Oh, Lord, what time is it? You think you're going to sneak inside me for a little snack. Sorry, it's too late to put anything in your mouth.

◇ ◇ ◇

So open the freezer and suck on an ice cube!

Cut this out and you know where it goes.
That's right, on the fridge.

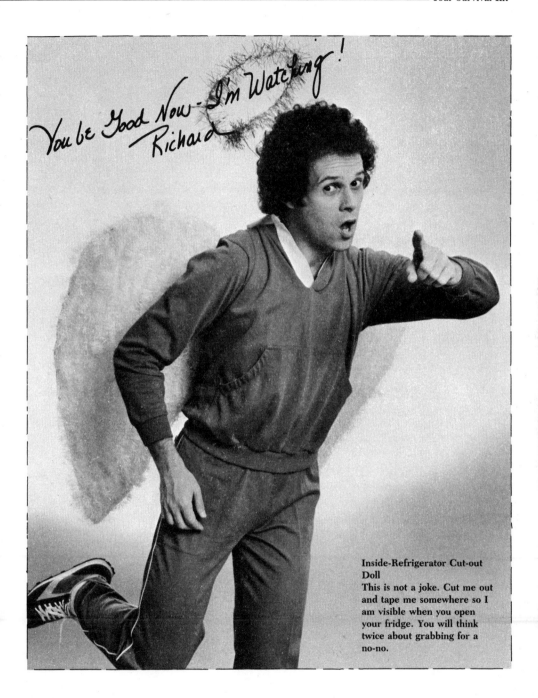

You be Good Now—I'm Watching!
Richard

Inside-Refrigerator Cut-out Doll
This is not a joke. Cut me out and tape me somewhere so I am visible when you open your fridge. You will think twice about grabbing for a no-no.

205

EMPTY-YOUR-PURSE TEST___

You think that because you cared enough to plunk down $7.95 for this book, you really care what you look like. You think, "This time I'm going to do it"; "This is really going to be the last diet book I ever buy," and all that.

Are you serious?

Let's see about it.

Ladies, empty your handbags on the dining-room table. Is there a Hershey kiss in your bra?

Gentlemen, I want everything on the table, too.

All right, let's take a good hard look.

Please check the appropriate answer.

1. Is there any chewing gum in the pile? Is it sugar-free?

2. Are there any hard candies? Life Savers have about three hundred calories in them. Even those little Freshen-up chewies you consume are fattening. Well, are there any there?

Yes___No___

3. How about chocolate-covered anythings?

Yes___No___

4. There aren't any candy bars—are there?

Yes___No___

5. How about packs of potato chips, Kraft caramels, pretzels, M&M's, or cheese and cracker packets?

Yes___No___

6. Is there any part of anything? Half a peanut butter and jelly sandwich wrapped in a napkin in case you get hungry later?

Yes___No___

7. Are there crumbs in the bottom of your handbag or in the lining of your pockets?

Yes___No___

SCORING

If you have any yes answers whatsoever, you should be ashamed of yourself! A person who is trying to lose weight should stay clear of anything that fits neatly into small areas like pockets or wallets (and then there's the old Milk Duds in the pants cuff trick—I used to do that myself).

YOU HAVE TWO CHOICES

1. Empty all that crap and never replace it, and think about your waistline next time you even consider putting a cough drop in your pocket.

2. Fall down on your knees, shake your head from left to right, maybe cry a few tears, and beg yourself for forgiveness!

MONTHLY GOAL SHEET___

At first, you will feel like you are back in first grade, but what's so bad about that? You were thinner back in first grade, remember?

The idea of writing down what you want out of this life is not such a bad idea. Any dream or goal you have first begins as a thought before becoming a reality, so why not jot it down? This technique, used by a lot of successful people, will give you direction, a clean-cut organized pattern, and believe me, you will never get bored because you'll be progressing and not spending time making a career out of eating.

Weight goals: I'd like to lose about ten more pounds this month; maybe I'll look into that new gym that just opened, but I'm not signing up for three years. I'll try it for a little while and see if it's a program I can live with.

Career goals: I plan to attend that series of nutrition lectures about protein structure and food. I've always wanted to learn more about what I eat anyway.

Domestic goals: This month I'll rearrange the furniture in the living room, save up for a new sofa, and paint one of the walls terracotta.

Health goals: I'm going to read up on medication so I can get to sleep faster without tossing and turning an hour every night.

Monetary goals: I'm going to watch my money flow this month and try to save two hundred dollars so I can buy some new clothes I need—a size down, I hope!

Cultural goals: I'm going to spend some time in the library and in that museum I've never been in and see a few movies I heard a lot about.

WHAT TO DO WHEN YOU'RE HAVING A SNACK ATTACK

What's a snack attack? You have the nerve to ask me what a snack attack is? It's when you get this urge . . . this tummy-trembling fit, when you feel like climbing the walls hoping to find a candy bar, a cookie, an "anything" to satisfy the hunger. We've all had them, and for some strange reason a Scarsdale carrot stick or a Pritikin string bean doesn't cut the mustard. (Speaking of mustard, I was once so crazed I ate a big family-size jar in about ten minutes—now, that's getting very desperate.)

Do I still get snack attacks even though I take good care of myself? Of course I do, but I have developed what is called "Snacker's Reasoning," a way of getting through to the cause before giving in and eating everything in sight.

Everyone knows that eating between meals means additional unnecessary volume, but no one seems to think about the fattening results while attacking food. Little dumb excuses come in handy and heavy when you feel like nibbling, for example:

> "I'm starving, and I behaved myself at breakfast, so I'll just have some of these very small, harmless cookies." (There is no such thing as a harmless cookie.)
>
> OR
>
> "So I'll eat this banana split and eat nothing else the rest of the day."

These are negative cop-outs; you are using the I.Q. of a baby flea. You must question yourself and wonder why you are feeling the need to feed your face. Remember, impulse can only mess up your pulse, not help it. That's why I'm going to teach you how Snacker's Reasoning can save your waistline.

Before grabbing at that bag of chips or even the healthiest of snacks, *stop* and look at your watch, find out what time it is. Come on, you can do this if you really want to. The whole key to holding snacking down to a minimum and controlling it forever is to be aware of what time these attacks strike. When do you get hungry?

● *Is it after breakfast and before lunch?* Why do you feel a food need? Come on, damn it, figure it out. Did you skip breakfast? No wonder you're hungry. You know, when you don't eat in the morning and get some life in your body, your energy level is shot! You get short-tempered, bored at work, and refuse to open your Master Charge bill until after you've had something to calm you down. If you did eat breakfast, then your stomach cannot be growling. It's your mind! You've got to have more guts— not more gut. Don't be afraid to question yourself and get to the bottom of the problem, not the bag of candy.

• *Do you start salivating after lunch and before dinner?* Why do you always feel more secure around the vending machine at about 3:00 P.M.? Did you skip lunch? Did you skip breakfast and lunch? Shame on you! Of course you're going to feel a little weak and want to eat. So again, I warn you to stop skipping meals and stay on your program. If you ate both meals, then why spoil dinner and the whole day? You've eaten correctly so far, your body is functioning properly, and the weight is coming off little by little. Why ruin all those positive things?

• *Does the Satan Snacker possess you after dinner and before bedtime?* Did you forget to eat dinner and decide to make up for the lost meal by rumbling through the fridge at 11:30 P.M.? Are you lonely? Do you often share your bed with Betty Crocker or Oscar Meyer? If you think eating a late dinner is a killer, what do you suppose a late snack is considered? The worst! Try to eat your dinner earlier, but don't skip it. If you followed your Live-It dinner menu, you shouldn't be hungry later on in the evening unless, of course, your emotions take over. Don't let them. Fight them with your strength and your reasoning. You can say no to that food. You want to lose this weight, don't you? You want to know finally how it feels to have control, don't you? Good. Now remember a

few minutes before you go night-night, mix up that water, lemon juice, and honey drink. It will put you right to sleep and you won't wake up with pepperoni and/or caramel-fudge-cake breath.

I understand you have tried to lose this weight before. You started off with fireworks and high energy and then you goofed and lost interest. That "goof" usually takes place at snacktime. Oh, sure, you can keep a bowl of cut-up vegetables in the fridge, but guess what, 90 percent of the time you are not at home when the attack hits. You're in a restaurant at an odd hour of the day, you're at a wedding, at the movies, in an airplane stuffing yourself with those salty dry-roasted peanuts. I don't know too many people who keep orange wedges and celery stalks hiding away in their coat pockets, do you? I didn't think so.

You cannot avoid all those times of the day when you are surrounded by food, so you'd better begin understanding yourself and your needs by practicing Snacker's Reasoning. Keep asking yourself, "Why am I feeling hungry?" "Why do I need another cup of coffee or another martini?" "Why am I going off my food plan when I know it's wrong?" When you are able to answer these questions by yourself, then snacking will never be a problem for you again.

Until you get that "inner strength" you're lacking, here are a few tips to help ease you off the snack road. Please try to reason with yourself first. I want to see you make it this time!

• Reach for a liquid instead of a solid. Liquids are easier to digest and tend to give you a "full feeling" immediately. On a day when you aren't in the mood for juice in the morning, have it an hour or so before lunch. If you skipped that iced tea at lunch, go ahead and drink it before suppertime. Don't knock a nice cold glass of water. It's about the best snack you can have.

● Chew a piece of gum. I feel the same way about gum as I do about soft drinks. What do you want to chew, a little sugar or an artificial sweetener that's supposed to reduce cavities but may contain cancer-causing agents? I don't think a stick of any kind of gum, once in a while, is going to kill you—besides, gum does keep your mouth busy.

● In many diet books is a list commonly known as free foods—foods you can eat "as much as you want of" and not interfere with weight loss. Nothing is free; celery sticks are volume and have to be digested just like any other foods. Don't be fooled by thinking you can drink all the coffee and tea you want, either.

● Keep referring to your food plan and always keep remembering not to duplicate foods. If you had a peach in the morning, then having another one a few hours later is senseless and unnecessary. With Snacker's Reasoning on your side, you should have no problem saying no.

THINGS TO REMEMBER WHEN YOU VISIT THE SUPERMARKET

Time to go shopping and pick up a few things for the house like Kleenex for the bedroom and toilet paper for the bathroom and—oh yes, food for the kitchen. You know all those animal, vegetable, and mineral products you stuff in the fridge and every inch of cabinet space? *Fact:* You will have a very difficult, almost impossible, time losing an ounce of fat if your whole environment is filled with items that are in mouth reach. You think restaurants are tough—you stock your kitchen like a restaurant! Little mints here, a dish of hard candy there, a freezer full of goodies just in case your husband brings the entire office building home for dinner.

You must start thinking of your kitchen as a savings account. You must deposit foods there that go along with your Live-It Program. If you keep fun food lying around everywhere, you're going to have a lot of difficulty saying no.

Here're a few tips to keep in mind the next time market day rolls around. If need be, cut this section out of the book and keep it in your wallet (next to the Live-It Program you're on). You'll end up with better products and better health—and those, my friends, are real savings.

Shopping for Breads

I know you love white fluffy bread. Who wasn't raised on sandwiches made with those heavenly slices? The saying of the eighties is now "the whiter the bread, the quicker you're dead." While that isn't true, there are better and healthier breads boasting 100 percent natural ingredients, natural fiber, and no chemicals added. They are a bit more expensive but the best choices for your body—no, they don't taste like sawdust, either—many contain a touch of raisin juice, oatmeal, wheat berries, and assorted grains. They're very tasty even without that bit of butter or jelly you're allowed.

Canned and Bottled Goods

Let's face it, all of us buy certain products

that are hard and sometimes impossible to prepare at home, like olives, pickles, ketch-up, etc. Now many products you use daily, such as juices, fruit, vegetables, soups, even meats, you also purchase in a can or bottle. Admit it, you're lazy and are taking the easy way out. You are not only paying for the string beans, but also the preservatives, dyes, chemicals, and a string of synthetics you don't want to know about. Another thing you don't realize is how long that can of sliced peaches has been sitting around. And since we're on the subject of sitting around, what do you do with all those fancy cans and jars and full-color labels? Throw them away—I knew it. There's more money you waste.

Special Canned and Bottled Goods

When a label says diet, low cal, low sodium, or instant, you are guaranteed that the price of these products instantly goes up. For some reason the diet items you buy off the shelves are usually pretty bad investments and suffer in taste. The sugar is taken out and chemicals are added. The salt is out and more chemicals are poured in. Flavor seems artificial and frankly, these foods are on the depressing side. These products do contain less calories, but remember, forget about counting!

Frozen-Food Section

You can buy anything frozen now, and I do mean anything. Vegetables with any favorite sauces can be ready in just a few minutes. Pizza, egg rolls, hero sandwiches, baked Alaska—foods and delicacies from every continent can be on your dinner table to-night! Like canned goods, everything you buy frozen can be prepared in your kitch-en—as I keep reminding you, go for fresh if you can. Frozen foods are more expensive. Remember, otherwise you are paying a lot extra for a bunch of people who work in a big factory cooking, packing, and freezing foods just for you. Isn't that nice?

Aisles to Avoid

Stay away from the cookie-and-cake aisle. Those Pepperidge Farm boxes can talk you into anything. Also watch out for that small section filled with foods from around the world. Smoked frogs' legs, octopus, and marinated pheasant eggs—forget them—imported fat is nothing to play around with. No fair looking at the new flavors of ice cream. Why tempt yourself, why suffer?

The Most Important Section in the Store

Yes, you guessed it—the produce section. Here's where you should start your shopping. For fresh salads, imaginative vegetable dishes, natural dessert—fruit. Here's the best place to spend your money. If you're not married try to meet someone in the produce business. Fresh does cost more—a glass of freshly squeezed orange juice costs a little more than bottled or imitation, but it's worth it.

If you are seeking the highest food quality for a certain amount of money, take some extra time and make wiser food decisions. You can afford to eat right. You can't afford not to.

THE LAST WORD

I wish I could pop out right here, at the end of my book, and help each one of you follow through on this program. I can't help feeling my words and good thoughts can guide you along.

I know you have suffered through overweight hell, and I don't want you to suffer anymore. It's not fair. We were not created to suffer through life. When I finally liked myself, inside and out, I stopped suffering and went out there to get all the things I wanted.

● You must do the same now.

● You must want to change and reshape your life.

● You must want to reach your goals as much as I want to help you get there.

● You must forget about all the bad experiences you've had with losing weight, gaining weight, and all those broken promises to yourself and others.

● Don't look back, only look forward.

● You must never forget you are a Very Special Individual.

● You are Unique.

● There isn't anyone else like You in the Whole Wide World.

● You are not Perfect.

● There is room for Improvement and Polish.

My Program can help make You a Better You. It can make You aware of your Potential. Give You strength and make You believe in yourself each and every day.

Now You have
all the ingredients
for your
Success Recipe—
Self-Love
A Positive Attitude
and
Determination.

Go Out There
and
Live-It.

If you need more motivation, please write:

Never Say Diet
P.O. Box 5403
Beverly Hills, CA 90210

Richard Simmons is now appearing on ABC-TV's *General Hospital*, America's most popular daytime series.

COMING IN JUNE 1982

Richard Simmons reveals phase II of his fat-fighting plan:
THE RICHARD SIMMONS NEVER-SAY-DIET COOKBOOK
including over 100 exclusive new recipes.
Available in a new Warner hardcover edition
(51-243, $15.95)

and from Elektra Records the
new Richard Simmons record album
REACH
Coming soon.

WATCH FOR THEM!!!